CORE
ANATOMY
ILLUSTRATED

CORE
ANATOMY
ILLUSTRATED

Ian Parkin MB ChB
Professor of Applied Clinical Anatomy, University of Dundee, and Royal College of Surgeons, Edinburgh; formerly Clinical Anatomist, University of Cambridge and Senior Lecturer in Anatomy, University of Birmingham

Bari M Logan MA FMA Hon MBIE MAMAA
Formerly University Prosector, Department of Anatomy, University of Cambridge; Prosector, Department of Anatomy, Royal College of Surgeons of England, London and Anatomical Preparator, Department of Human Morphology, University of Nottingham Medical School

Mark J McCarthy MB ChB PhD FRCS (Eng) FRCS (Edin)
Consultant Vascular Surgeon and Honorary Senior Lecturer, Department of Vascular and Endovascular Surgery, Leicester Royal Infirmary

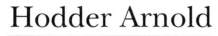

Hodder Arnold

A MEMBER OF THE HODDER HEADLINE GROUP

CRC Press
Taylor & Francis Group
6000 Broken Sound Parkway NW, Suite 300
Boca Raton, FL 33487-2742

© 2017 by Taylor & Francis Group, LLC
CRC Press is an imprint of Taylor & Francis Group, an Informa business

No claim to original U.S. Government works

Printed on acid-free paper
Version Date: 20170126

International Standard Book Number-13: 978-0-340-80918-1 (Hardback)

Visit the Taylor & Francis Web site at
http://www.taylorandfrancis.com

and the CRC Press Web site at
http://www.crcpress.com

Contents

PART IV The Thorax

PART V The Abdomen

PART VI The Male and Female Pelvis

Dedications

To my dear wife, my family and my friends who have supported me unfailingly throughout the ups and downs of this project. Also to my colleagues past and present, anatomical, educational, technical and secretarial without whom I would not have learned enough to get past the first page.
Ian Parkin

To Angie James, for bringing me back to life, and to my son Robert Logan.
Bari Logan

To my dearest wife, Lucy and my wonderful children Madelyne, Joseph and Oscar. I also dedicate this book to the loving memory of my father, Anthony McCarthy.
Mark McCarthy

Foreword

It is incontrovertible that, in recent years, most undergraduate and postgraduate medical curricula in this country and elsewhere have been so designed as to result in a progressive and significant reduction in the time allocated to the study of topographical anatomy. In large measure this has been due to the competing demands exercised by a variety of other disciplines and the consequent need to reassign educational priorities.

Traditional textbooks of anatomy, with their emphasis on topographical details and their relative lack of clinically-pertinent information are thus largely inappropriate to present-day undergraduate medical curricula.

The publication of **Core Anatomy – Illustrated** is therefore a timely and valuable intervention. The book addresses the requirements of the new curricula in a most effective manner.

Taking advantage of their vast experience in teaching and examining medical undergraduates and postgraduates, the authors have, in my view, struck a very satisfactory and harmonious balance between the amount of topographical anatomical information on the one hand, and its clinical relevance on the other. In so doing they have succeeded in defining the scope of core anatomical knowledge.

The book is well-organized and the layout is exemplary. The text is written in an admirably lucid and concise style, making the subject matter readily assimilable. The plentiful illustrations (in particular, the photographs of dissections) are of superlative quality and do much to enhance the book.

Professor Parkin and his colleagues Messrs Logan and McCarthy are to be generously applauded for their imaginativeness in conceiving of this volume, and for presenting the subject matter in an unambiguous manner.

I believe that the primary readership for whom this book is intended, namely undergraduate medical and dental students, postgraduate surgical trainees and students in paramedical fields, will benefit considerably from this very readable and useful book.

I wish the book every success.

Professor Vishy Mahadevan MBBS PhD FRCSEd (Hon) FDSRCSEng FRCS
Barbers' Company Reader in Anatomy & Head of Surgical Anatomy
The Royal College of Surgeons of England, London, UK

Acknowledgements

The authors are most grateful to the following:

For continued encouragement to produce this book and allowing the use of facilities, Professor Bill Harris, Department of Anatomy, University of Cambridge, Cambridge, UK.

For photographs, digital expertise and advice, Mr Adrian Newman, Mr Ian Bolton and Mr John Bashford, Anatomy Visua Media Group, Department of Anatomy, University of Cambridge, Cambridge, UK.

Emily Evans at Medical Illustration for her line drawings.

Georgina Bentliff, Heather Smith, Joanna Koster, Clare Weber, Sara Purdy, Jane Tod, Clare Patterson and all the team at Hodder Arnold Health Sciences for their help and advice during the preparation of this book.

Furthermore, the illustrations, which are vital to this textbook, would not have been possible without the extreme generosity of those members of the public who bequeathed their bodies for medical education and research.

Dissection/anatomical preparation credits

The following individuals are to be credited for their skilled work in preparing the anatomical material illustrated in this book:

Mrs C Bester	– 151D, 159B
Dr N Borley	– 61B
Ms M Lazenby	– 71AB, 109D, 111BC, 113C
Bari M Logan	– 15B, 17ABC, 21ABCD, 23ABCDE, 25ABCD, 27ABCD, 29ABC, 31ABCDEF, 33ABCDEF, 35ABCDE, 37ABCDEF, 39ABCDE, 41ABCD, 43AB, 45ABCDEFG, 47ABCD, 49ABC, 51ABCD, 53ABC, 55AB, 57ABC, 59A, 61A, 65A, 67A, 69ABC, 71C, 73ABCD, 75ACD, 77ABC, 79ABCD, 81ABCDE, 83ABCD, 87AB, 89B, 91ABCD, 93ABCD, 95ABC, 97AB, 99ABC, 101B, 105AB, 109BC, 113B, 115AB, 117A, 119A, 121A, 123B, 125A, 129AB, 133AC, 135A, 137ABC, 139B, 143AB, 145ABC, 147AB, 151A, 153AB, 155A, 157AB, 161A, 163A, 165ABC
Ms L Nearn	– 111A, 113A, 151BC, 159C, 161B, 163BC
Mr M Watson	– 159A
Ms L Whithead	– 109A, 133B, 139A, 141AB

Preface

Since the early 1990s, major changes have taken place in the way human anatomy is taught within educational institutions throughout the world.

Essentially these changes may be attributed to the fact that much of the new and exciting, ground breaking research in topographical anatomy was done two hundred to four hundred years ago. Anatomists have moved away from dedicated gross anatomical research and teaching roles towards the scientific disciplines of genetics or cellular, molecular and neuro-biology, and development. This wealth of new knowledge that is equally essential to the effective practice of any health professional, has led to a substantial reduction in course curricula hours dedicated to the learning of anatomy.

In parallel, there has been a long over due re-appraisal of teaching and learning methodology culminating in an unfortunate and widespread abandonment of practical, cadaver dissection classes in favour of the use of prosections, but with the exciting inclusion of small-group and problem-solving tutorials, or interactive multimedia computer-aided learning. Medical and paramedical education must no longer be divided into undergraduate and postgraduate sections, but seen as a continuum which builds and reinforces knowledge as it is required in practice.

The mainstay of these educational developments has been the notion of 'core' courses, usually supplemented by additional, student-selected course components. 'Core' is considered to be a course content offering the most essential, relevant basic knowledge required for safe practice. However, 'core' is open to interpretation and opinion, from institution to institution, and between different academics. Consequently, with our combined experience of teaching and assessing gross human anatomy, and of providing highly detailed anatomical material for both practical classes and museum study, we have created this book of what we consider to be 'core anatomy': the relevant, basic but essential, anatomy required for safe, effective clinical practice, whether as a student or as a junior, postgraduate trainee.

The book intends to be brief, concise and very much to the point. Although the text contains only the anatomy that is felt to be functionally or clinically important, it is at sufficient depth to facilitate understanding and, therefore, deeper learning. Its concentration may be overwhelming to the first-time reader, but its aim is to review anatomy in preparation for all aspects of clinical work. The content has been designed to fit with, and relate to the spread of illustrations opposite. Therefore it follows a tight regional and 'visible' pattern that may appear at odds with a more systemic or systematic approach.

We hope the book will be well used and enjoyed. It is not 'set in stone', we expect the debate on 'core' to continue and look forward to comments from our anatomy colleagues on what we should have left out, and what we should have included. We will listen to, and take heed of these, but hope that our efforts overall are seen to be contributing a positive move towards supporting and continuing the teaching of human gross anatomy.

Ian Parkin, Bari Logan and Mark McCarthy
2007

How to use this book

The most effective method of learning any subject is to see its relevance, to work with it and to apply it. This book invites the reader to work with the anatomy, cross-referencing between the text page and the accompanying illustrations, or vice-versa. Each section should be seen and used as a whole entity.

Throughout the book the anatomical illustrations are shown on the right-hand page of each double-page spread, with an explanatory key beneath. Numbering in the key is coloured according to the importance of each anatomical structure. Core anatomical structures are shown with a coloured number, and the first reference to them in the text is also highlighted in colour. When a number is given in black in the key, this indicates a non-core anatomical structure; these are illustrated in order to provide the reader with more detailed reference or orientation points. Underneath this key is a list showing which illustration(s) each number appears on. Clinical information is highlighted in the text by a sans serif font with a pointing-hand icon in the margin as a simple but effective method to draw the reader's eye.

Where possible groups of muscles have been combined functionally and the nerve supply to the whole group is given at the end of the appropriate paragraph or section. The root value of the major or clinically important nerves appears in parentheses after the nerve. For example, this sentence follows the paragraph on quadriceps: 'The femoral nerve (L2,3,4) supplies all these muscles (knee jerk L3,4).' Where such grouping is not possible, the nerve supply (and root value if considered relevant) follows each muscle.

When referring to vertebral levels or to the spinal nerves that contribute to peripheral nerves (i.e. the root value), the accepted abbreviations have been used: cervical (C); thoracic (T); lumbar (L); sacral (S). Therefore, although 'C6' can refer to the sixth cervical vertebra or to the sixth cervical spinal nerve the context will make the choice completely obvious. Cranial nerves are indicated by the usual practice of Roman numerals.

Orientation symbols have been placed in a corner of each illustration, indicating Superior (S), Inferior (I), Right (R), Left (L), Posterior (P), Anterior (A), Medial (M), Lateral (Lat), Dorsal (Dor), Plantar (Plan), Distal (D), Proximal (Prox) and Palmar (Pal).

Terminology

Terminology normally conforms to the International Anatomical Terminology – Terminologia Anatomica – created in 1998 by the Federative Committee on Anatomical Terminology (FCAT) and approved by the 56 member Associations of the International Federation of Associations of Anatomists (IFAA). However, the text is for medical students and junior doctors who will be working alongside clinicians who may, themselves, be using a more familiar terminology. Therefore, such terminology has been included, and where it is shorter and easier to read it has become the primary one. The textboxes include both terminologies. Similarly, eponymous terminology has been included if in common use.

For example: The Greek adjective 'peroneal' is now replaced by the Latin 'fibular' for various muscles, vessels, nerves and structures of the lower limb, e.g. fibularis tertius instead of peroneus tertius; fibular artery instead of peroneal artery; common fibular nerve instead of common peroneal nerve. In this book, the term peroneal is included in parentheses to help identify changes for those referring to other older texts, e.g. common fibular (peroneal) nerve. Also note that flexor accessorius is known as quadratus plantae. The adrenal gland is referred to as suprarenal, but the shorter term vas or vas deferens has been retained instead of ductus deferens.

Parts of the body

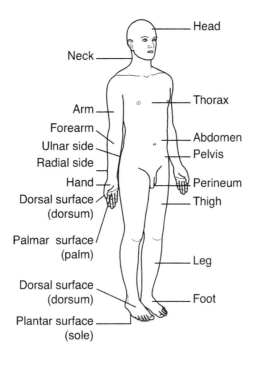

Anatomical planes

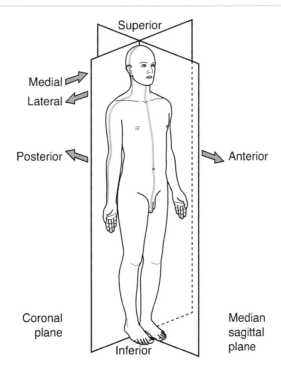

Figures reproduced from McMinn RMH, Gaddum-Rosse P, Hutchings RT, Logan BM (1995) *McMinn's Functional and Clinical Anatomy*. London: Mosby-Wolfe.

Movements of the upper limb

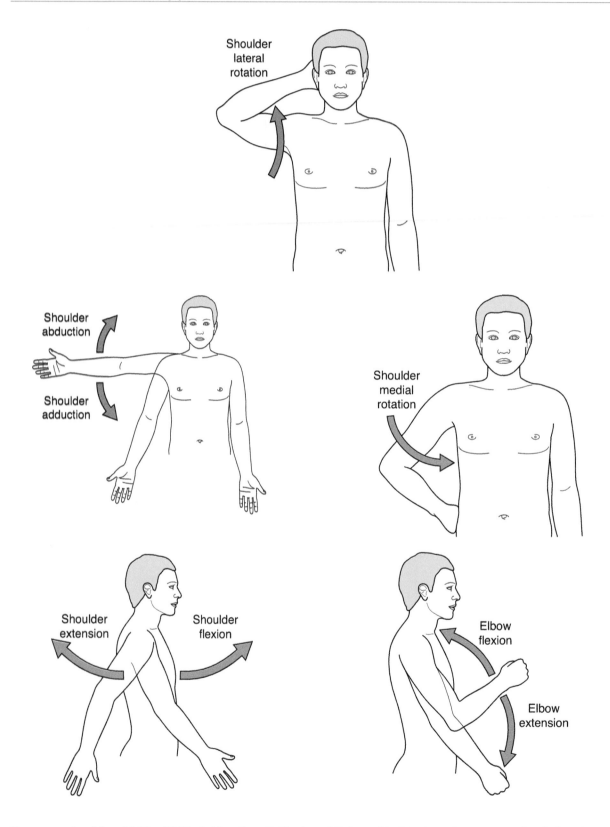

Figures reproduced from McMinn RMH, Gaddum-Rosse P, Hutchings RT, Logan BM (1995) *McMinn's Functional and Clinical Anatomy*. London: Mosby-Wolfe.

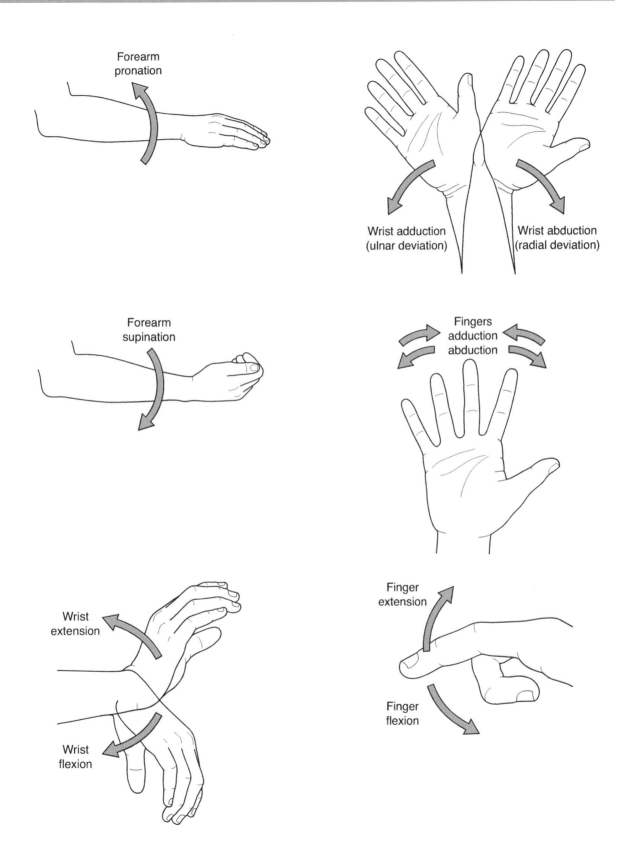

Forearm pronation

Wrist adduction (ulnar deviation)

Wrist abduction (radial deviation)

Forearm supination

Fingers adduction abduction

Wrist extension

Wrist flexion

Finger extension

Finger flexion

Figures reproduced from McMinn RMH, Gaddum-Rosse P, Hutchings RT, Logan BM (1995) *McMinn's Functional and Clinical Anatomy*. London: Mosby-Wolfe.

Movements of the trunk and lower limb

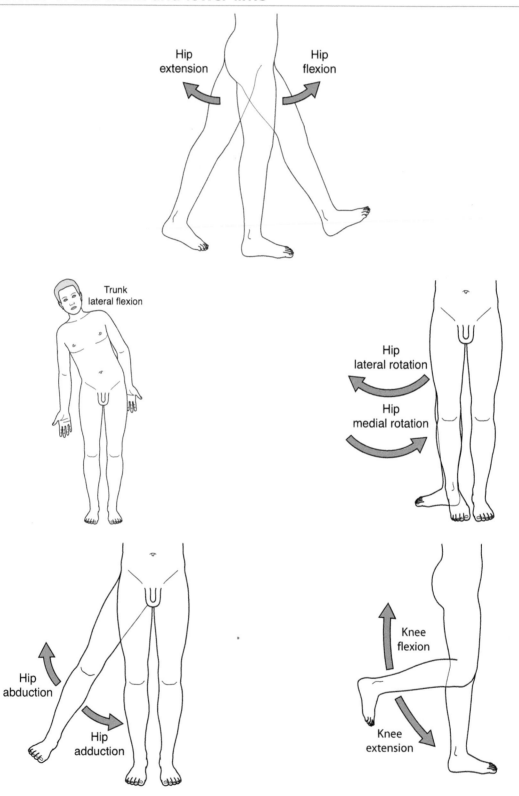

Figures reproduced from McMinn RMH, Gaddum-Rosse P, Hutchings RT, Logan BM (1995) *McMinn's Functional and Clinical Anatomy*. London: Mosby-Wolfe.

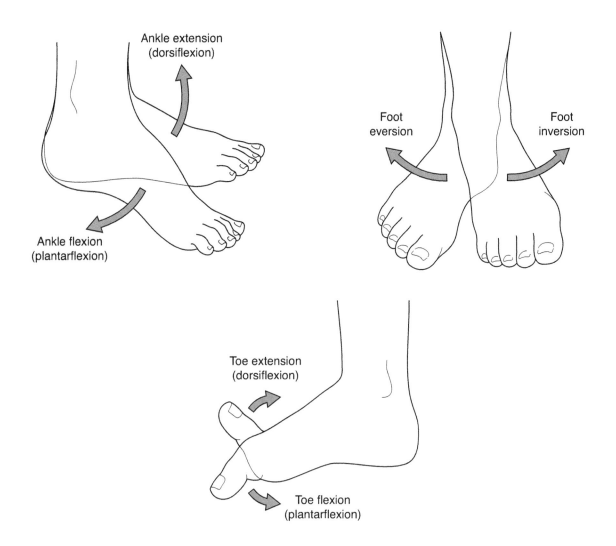

Figures reproduced from McMinn RMH, Gaddum-Rosse P, Hutchings RT, Logan BM (1995) *McMinn's Functional and Clinical Anatomy.* London: Mosby-Wolfe.

Movements: basic terminology

Abduction	– movement away from the midline of the body
Adduction	– movement toward the midline of the body
Eversion	– turning outward
Inversion	– turning inward
Flexion	– bending
Extension	– extending or stretching, straightening out
Pronation	– twisting or turning of bones over one another
Supination	– untwisting bones over one another
	[terms specific to the forearm bones, radius and ulna]
Rotation	– twisting in the long axis of a bone

Part I

The Skeleton

Skeleton, bones of upper limb

Bones

Bones are essentially for movement, being a system of supportive levers connected by joints that usually have a cartilaginous component. Bones may be protective, but fracture may cause soft tissue damage. Bone is a mineral store (calcium, phosphate) and is for haemopoiesis (all bones in infants, but only flat bones in adults). Therefore, they must be dynamic and ever changing, remodelling to fulfil these functions and cope with altered stresses or loads. For similar reasons bones must be vascular, and fracture may cause considerable blood loss. The high demands and high turnover make bones susceptible to poor nutrition. Bones have the general structure of a compact outer 'case', supported by a series of internal tie-bars of cancellous bone. They are covered by periosteum, with outer fibrous and inner cellular layers.

Cartilage

Cartilage is largely avascular and is tough, flexible and light. Perichondrium covers cartilage as periosteum covers bone. Cartilage is typified by cells lying in lacunae within a connective tissue matrix. There are three types of cartilage. Hyaline cartilage has a smooth, glassy appearance. It forms the costal cartilages (1) and epiphyseal growth plates, and lines synovial joints as friction-free, articular cartilage (no perichondrium on the joint surfaces). Bones joined to bones by short pieces of hyaline cartilage are synchondroses or primary cartilaginous joints, e.g. first rib (2) to manubrium. Fibrocartilage has cells in a fibrous matrix. It is shock absorptive and resilient, to withstand shearing. Joints that contain fibrocartilage are symphyses or secondary cartilaginous joints, e.g. joints in the midline of the body, manubriosternal joint (3), vertebral discs (4) and pubic symphysis (5). Elastic cartilage has cells in a matrix of elastic fibres. It is springy and returns to its original position after displacement.

Axial skeleton

The axial skeleton consists of: skull (6); mandible (7); sternum (8); ribs (9); and vertebrae (10).

Appendicular skeleton

The appendicular skeleton consists of: pelvic girdle (hip bones (11) and sacrum (12)); pectoral girdle – scapula (13) and clavicle (14); humerus (15), radius (16), ulna (17); femur (18), tibia (19), fibula (20); carpus (21) and metacarpals (22); tarsus (23) and metatarsals (24); and phalanges (25).

Upper limb bones

The clavicle has a blunt, quadrangular medial end, which forms the sternoclavicular joint (26), the main ligament of which runs from the clavicle to the first costal cartilage – the costoclavicular ligament. It is the true attachment of the upper limb and pectoral girdle to the rest of the body. As it lies just lateral to the joint it acts as a pivotal point, and thus the movements of the sternoclavicular joint may be regarded as of a ball and socket joint.

The lateral end of the clavicle forms the acromioclavicular joint (27) with the acromion (28) of the scapula. The joint is stabilized by the strong coracoclavicular ligament, which has two segments (conoid and trapezoid) and firmly binds the clavicle to the underlying coracoid process (29). Both sternoclavicular and acromioclavicular joints are synovial but atypical – they have fibrocartilage on the articular surfaces and also have intracapsular discs. If the clavicle is fractured following direct trauma or a fall on the extended limb it tends to fracture between the lateral third and medial two-thirds. The weight of the upper limb pulls the lateral segment of the clavicle inferiorly.

The first metacarpal bone (30) has a saddle-shaped proximal end to provide a more freely mobile carpometacarpal joint, quite different from the others. It rotates to allow the movement of opposition of the terminal pulp (pad) of the thumb to that of the little finger. The thumb has two phalanges whereas the other digits have three. The metacarpophalangeal joints allow abduction and adduction, and flexion and extension. The combination of these four movements gives circumduction but no rotation. The interphalangeal joints allow only hinge movement and thus have strong collateral ligaments.

The anatomical 'snuff box' lies at the base of the thumb lateral to the tendon of extensor pollicis longus, between it and the tendons of abductor longus and extensor brevis. The radial artery passes across the floor of the 'snuff box', and tenderness here suggests scaphoid (31) fracture.

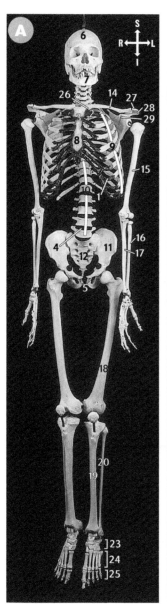
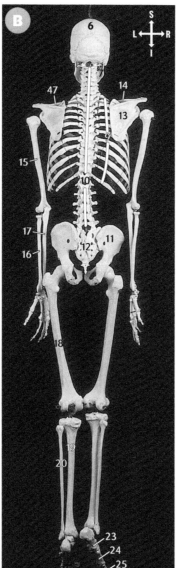
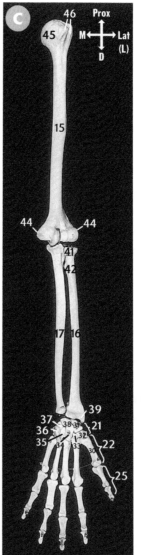
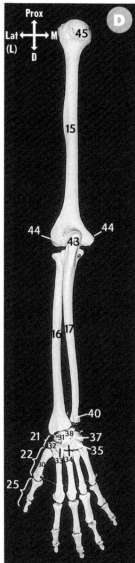

A **Skeleton (from the front)**
B **Skeleton (from behind)**
C **Bones of the upper limb (from the front)**
D **Bones of the upper limb (from behind)**

1 Costal cartilages (hyaline cartilage)	12 Sacrum	24 Metatarsal bones
2 First costal cartilage	13 Scapula	25 Phalanges
3 Manubriosternal joint and sternal angle	14 Clavicle	26 Sternoclavicular joint
	15 Humerus	27 Acromioclavicular joint
4 Intervertebral disc	16 Radius	28 Acromion of scapula
5 Pubic symphysis	17 Ulna	29 Coracoid process of scapula
6 Skull	18 Femur	30 First metacarpal bone
7 Mandible	19 Tibia	31 Scaphoid bone
8 Sternum	20 Fibula	32 Trapezium
9 Ribs	21 Carpal bones	33 Trapezoid
10 Vertebrae	22 Metacarpal bones	34 Capitate
11 Hip bone	23 Tarsal bones	35 Hamate

36 Pisiform	42 Tuberosity of radius
37 Triquetral	43 Olecranon of ulna
38 Lunate	44 Epicondyles
39 Styloid process of radius	45 Head of humerus
40 Styloid process of ulna	46 Tuberosities of humerus
41 Head of radius	47 Spine of scapula

Location of numbers: 1A; 2A; 3A; 4A; 5A; 6AB; 7A; 8A; 9AB; 10AB; 11AB; 12AB; 13B; 14AB; 15ABCD; 16ABCD; 17ABCD; 18AB; 19AB; 20AB; 21CD; 22CD; 23AB; 24AB; 25ABCD; 26A; 27A; 28A; 29A; 30CD; 31CD; 32CD; 33CD; 34CD; 35CD; 36C; 37CD; 38CD; 39C; 40D; 41C; 42C; 43D; 44CD; 45CD; 46C; 47B.

Skeleton of pelvis and lower limb, popliteal fossa, foot ligaments

The pelvic girdle is formed by the hip bones (1) articulating with each other and with the sacrum (2).

The sacro-iliac joints (3) are synovial with a fibrous capsule supported by strong anterior, posterior and intra-articular ligaments. Movement is limited. The ligaments relax a little during pregnancy, allowing a wider pelvis for delivery, but possibly causing back pain. (also caused by arthritis of the joints). The body weight tends to tilt the upper sacrum down and forward, but the lower sacrum is prevented from consequently swivelling up and backward by the sacrotuberous (4) and sacrospinous (5) ligaments. The former passes to the ischial tuberosity from the posterior aspects of the ilium, sacrum and coccyx, lying external to the sacrospinous ligament that passes to the ischial spine from a smaller, sacral origin. The greater sciatic foramen (6) transmits nerves and vessels from the pelvis to the buttock. The lesser sciatic foramen (7) is inferior to the sacrospinous ligament, therefore inferior to the pelvic floor. Nerves and vessels passing through it enter the perineum.

The pubic symphysis (8) is a fibrocartilaginous joint between the bodies of the two pubic bones (9). It is supported by ligaments, has little movement and aids shock absorption during walking.

The pelvic brim, or entry into the true pelvis, is bounded by the pubic symphysis, pubic crest (10), superior pubic ramus with its pectineal line (11), the arcuate line (12) and the sacral promontory (13). It faces anteriorly so that the pubic tubercles (14) are in the same vertical (coronal) plane as the anterior superior iliac spines (15) but in the same horizontal plane as the ischial spines (16). The pelvic outlet is bounded by the coccyx (17), ischial tuberosities (18), ischiopubic rami (19) and pubic symphysis. The outlet faces inferiorly and is for the passage of the urethra and anal canal, and vagina in the female.

The female pelvis must be capable of childbirth; therefore, it is lighter, wider and more rounded than the male pelvis, which has a more 'closed' appearance, particularly at the outlet. To achieve the wider female pelvis: the subpubic angle between the ischiopubic rami is wider; superior pubic rami are longer than the acetabular diameter; ischial spines do not encroach upon the outlet; and the pelvic brim is wider in the transverse direction than anteroposteriorly.

Popliteal fossa

The popliteal fossa (20) lies behind the knee joint between semitendinosus/semimembranosus and biceps femoris superiorly and the two heads of gastrocnemius inferiorly. In the fossa, the sciatic nerve divides into the tibial and common fibular (peroneal) nerves. The superficial femoral artery and vein pass through the adductor hiatus to become the popliteal vessels within the fossa, with the artery next to the bone and knee joint capsule. The popliteal artery is at risk in fractures and dislocations of the knee, resulting in intimal tears and possible limb ischaemia. The tibial nerve lies superficial to the popliteal vein as it runs inferiorly to supply the muscles in the posterior compartments of the leg. The common fibular (peroneal) nerve lies next to the tendon of semitendinosus, passes to the neck of the fibula (where the nerve is at risk of injury from fibula fractures) and winds around it.

The popliteal artery divides into the anterior tibial artery and the tibioperoneal trunk. The anterior tibial passes above the interosseous membrane to join the deep fibular (peroneal) nerve. The tibioperoneal trunk divides into the posterior tibial artery, which runs with the nerve of the same name and fibular (peroneal) artery, which supplies the fibular muscles.

Foot ligaments

Many ligaments hold the tarsal and metatarsal bones together. The fibrocartilage spring ligament (plantar calcaneonavicular) supports the head of the talus (40) by passing from the sustentaculum tali (41) to the navicular (42). The long and short plantar ligaments pass from the calcaneus (43) to the cuboid (44). The short ligament attaches proximal to the groove for fibularis (peroneus) longus (45), the long ligament attaches distally, converting the groove into a canal. On the dorsum of the foot, the bifurcate ligament supports the arch from above and passes in two directions, from calcaneus to cuboid and calcaneus to navicular.

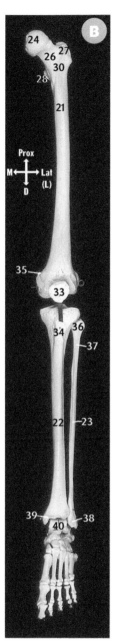

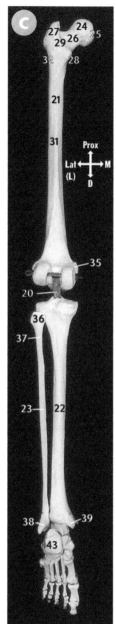

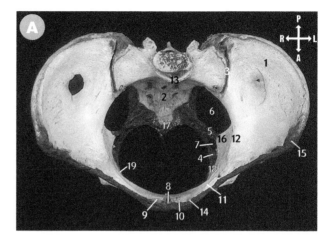

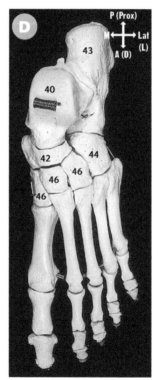

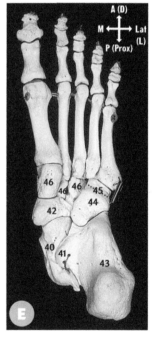

A Articulated pelvis (from above)
B Bones of the lower limb (from the front)
C Bones of the lower limb (from behind)

D Bones of the foot, dorsal surface (from above)
E Bones of the foot, plantar surface (from below)

1	Hip bone	14	Pubic tubercle
2	Sacrum	15	Anterior superior iliac spine
3	Sacro-iliac joint	16	Ischial spine
4	Sacrotuberous ligament	17	Coccyx
5	Sacrospinous ligament	18	Ischial tuberosity
6	Greater sciatic foramen	19	Ischiopubic ramus
7	Lesser sciatic foramen	20	Position of popliteal fossa
8	Pubic symphysis	21	Femur
9	Body of pubic bone	22	Tibia
10	Pubic crest	23	Fibula
11	Pectineal line	24	Head of femur
12	Arcuate line	25	Fovea for ligament of head of femur
13	Promontory of sacrum		

26	Neck of femur	39	Medial malleolus of tibia
27	Greater trochanter	40	Talus
28	Lesser trochanter	41	Sustentaculum tali of calcaneus
29	Intertrochanteric crest	42	Navicular
30	Intertrochanteric line	43	Calcaneus
31	Linea aspera	44	Cuboid
32	Gluteal tuberosity	45	Groove for fibularis (peroneus) longus
33	Patella	46	Cuneiforms (lateral, intermediate, medial)
34	Tuberosity of tibia		
35	Adductor tubercle of femur		
36	Head of fibula		
37	Neck of fibula		
38	Lateral malleolus of fibula		

Location of numbers: 1A; 2A; 3A; 4A; 5A; 6A; 7A; 8A; 9A; 10A; 11A; 12A; 13A; 14A; 15A; 16A; 17A; 18A; 19A; 20C; 21BC; 22BC; 23BC; 24BC; 25C; 26BC; 27BC; 28BC; 29C; 30B; 31C; 32C; 33B; 34B; 35BC; 36BC; 37BC; 38BC; 39BC; 40BDE; 41E; 42DE; 43CDE; 44DE; 45E; 46DE.

Part II

The Vertebral Column

Individual vertebrae, lateral view of vertebral column, curvatures

The vertebral column supports the weight of the body as well as containing the spinal cord and emerging spinal nerves. It must be strong but flexible, therefore, it is composed of a series of vertebrae, with limited movement available between consecutive vertebrae. A typical vertebra has a body (1), two pedicles (2) and two laminae (3), which fuse at the spinous process (4), and two transverse processes (5). The inferior and superior (6) articular facets form synovial joints with equivalent facets on the vertebra above and below.

There are seven cervical, twelve thoracic and five lumbar vertebrae. The sacrum and coccyx are formed by fused vertebrae: five in the sacrum, three or four in the coccyx. At birth, the vertebral column shows the primary curvature, concave anteriorly. But as the infant lifts its head, then stands up to walk, secondary curvatures, concave posteriorly, develop in the cervical and lumbar regions.

Between two consecutive vertebral bodies is an intervertebral disc (7), which has an annulus of fibrocartilage enclosing a hygroscopic jelly, the nucleus pulposus. The discs hold the bodies together and provide shock absorption. Their deformation allows limited movement, but the direction of that movement is dictated by the shape of the articular facets. The whole vertebral column is also supported by ligaments:

- anterior longitudinal – anterior to the bodies and discs
- posterior longitudinal – attached to the posterior aspects of the discs and edges of the bodies
- inter-transverse and inter-spinous – between the transverse processes and between the spines, respectively
- supraspinous – joining the tips of the spines
- elastic ligamenta flava – between the laminae.

The typical cervical vertebra has a relatively small but wide vertebral body (8). The edges of the upper surface are turned upward to form joints with the down-turned edges of the inferior surface of the vertebra above. These joints may develop a painful arthritis (cervical spondylitis). The transverse processes have foramina (9), which transmit the vertebral artery. The C7 spine is palpable as the vertebra prominens.

The atlas (C1) does not have a body, but has two lateral masses (10) linked by a short anterior arch and a long posterior arch. The upper facets are concave ovals for articulation with the skull, allowing much of the flexion/extension of the head and neck. The inferior facets are flat and round. They articulate with the axis (C2) and allow rotation around the odontoid peg (dens) (11), which arises from the axis and lies behind the anterior arch of the atlas. Further ligaments bind the atlas and axis to each other as well as to the skull. Fracture of the odontoid peg can result in spinal cord damage and death. Likewise, a 'hangman's fracture' is the result of hyperextension of the cervical spine which leads to fracture of the pedicle of C2.

The thoracic vertebrae have bodies that are longer anteroposteriorly, and their spinous processes are long and point downward. The bodies and transverse processes show facets for the ribs. The lumbar vertebrae have large, wide, weight-bearing bodies and thick, quadrangular spinous processes.

The vertebral column is held upright by erector spinae, a thick multilayered column of muscle on each side, posteriorly. Anteriorly and laterally the abdominal wall muscles are also important for vertebral column support and movement. Erector spinae has multiple insertions, and it can extend, rotate and flex laterally. The multiple ligament and muscle insertions are all sites susceptible to strain, giving rise to immediate local back pain, aggravated by associated muscle spasm. Discs deteriorate with age and the nucleus may rupture or prolapse through the annulus to press onto the spinal cord or, more commonly onto a spinal nerve on its way to emerge from an intervertebral foramen (12).

There are valveless veins within the vertebral bodies that allow the metastatic spread of tumour into the bodies themselves, e.g. from prostatic, lung and breast cancers.

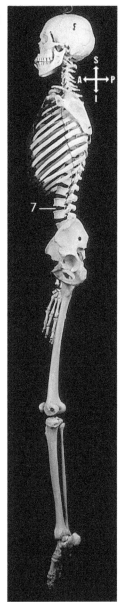

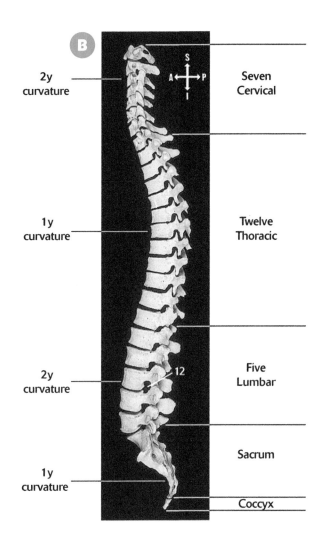

2y curvature

1y curvature

2y curvature

1y curvature

Seven Cervical

Twelve Thoracic

Five Lumbar

Sacrum

Coccyx

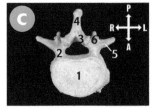

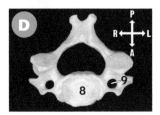

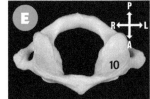

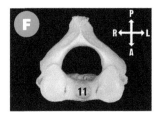

A   Skeleton with bones of the left upper and lower limb removed (from the left)
B   Bones of the vertebral column (from the left)
C   Lumbar vertebra (from above)

D   Cervical vertebra (from above)
E   Atlas (first cervical vertebra) (from above)
F   Axis (second cervical vertebra) (from above)

1	Body of lumbar vertebra	5	Transverse process of lumbar vertebra
2	Pedicle of lumbar vertebra	6	Superior articular facet of lumbar vertebra
3	Lamina of lumbar vertebra	7	Position of intervertebral disc
4	Spinous process of lumbar vertebra		

8	Body of cervical vertebra
9	Transverse foramen of cervical vertebra
10	Lateral mass of atlas, first cervical vertebra with superior articular

facet for the occipital condyle of skull
11   Odontoid peg (dens) of axis, the second cervical vertebra
12   Intervertebral foramen

Location of numbers: 1C; 2C; 3C; 4C; 5C; 6C; 7A; 8D; 9D; 10E; 11F; 12B.

Vertebral column, spinal cord, meninges, emerging nerves

Following removal of the overlying skin, erector spinae muscles, vertebral laminae and spines, the spinal cord is visible from behind.

The spinal cord (1) commences at the foramen magnum (2) as a continuation of the medulla (3). In the adult it usually ends (4) at the L1/2 disc, but at L2/3 in the infant.

The vertebral canal is lined by dura mater (5), forming a dural sac that ends at S2. The sac is lined by arachnoid mater. The spinal cord, closely covered by pia mater, is suspended in cerebrospinal fluid in the subarachnoid space. A flange of pia on each side sends fine denticulate ligaments to anchor the cord, via the arachnoid, to the overlying dural sac. These, and the filum terminale, a fibrous extension of the cord running all the way to the coccyx, prevent excessive movement of the cord. There is an epidural (potential) space (6) containing fat and a plexus of valveless veins between the dura and the bone, and ligaments of the vertebral canal. This potential space is used in anaesthesia. Infiltration of local anaesthetic agents results in temporary anaesthesia of the nerves below, therefore allowing surgical procedures to be undertaken for childbirth to take place. A lumbar puncture to collect a sample of cerebrospinal fluid (CSF) must be done below L1/2 to avoid cord damage. The usual site is L3/4.

The spinal cord is usually supplied by one anterior and two posterior arteries (7), which freely anastomose with each other and are variably augmented by additional arteries entering the intervertebral foramina. Loss of these, say in the thoracic or lumbar region following aortic aneurysm, may cause cord ischaemia.

Dorsal rootlets (8), which are sensory, emerge from the cord and combine with the motor, ventral rootlets (9) to form the mixed spinal nerves (10). The mixed spinal nerves, still encased in pia, arachnoid and dura mater emerge from each intervertebral foramen, where a swelling, the dorsal root ganglion (11), formed by clusters of sensory cell bodies, is visible on the nerve. Emerging nerves are named in relation to the vertebrae. Cervical (C) spinal nerves C1–7 emerge above cervical vertebrae C1–7. Then the pattern changes. The C8 nerve emerges inferior to C7 vertebra. All nerves then emerge inferior to the vertebra which gives the name, e.g. thoracic (T)1 below vertebra T1, lumbar (L)1 below vertebra L1, sacral (S)1 below S1 vertebra and so on.

Spinal cord segments are named after the nerve that arises from them. As the cord ends at L1/2 the remaining lumbar, sacral and coccygeal nerves form a bundle of nerves, the cauda equina (12), as they pass to the intervertebral foramina through which they leave the canal. Consequently spinal cord segments lie progressively higher in the vertebral canal. The segments giving rise to nerves C1–8 lie opposite the C1–7 vertebrae. Those giving rise to nerves T1–12 lie opposite vertebrae T1–10, whereas the segments giving rise to the five lumbar, five sacral, and coccygeal nerves lie opposite vertebrae T11–12 and L1.

Having emerged from the intervertebral foramina and the dural sheath, the spinal nerves receive postganglionic sympathetic fibres. Each nerve then divides into a dorsal ramus, to supply skin and muscle segmentally in the posterior midline, and a ventral ramus. These ventral rami (13) form the cervical (C1–4), brachial (C5–T1) and lumbosacral (L4–5 S1–4) plexuses as well as named nerves (e.g. phrenic), and the intercostal nerves. The extra cell bodies and nerves required for upper and lower limb function result in the cervical and lumbar enlargements of the spinal cord.

The lumbar nerves emerge from the intervertebral foramina in a notch between the pedicle and vertebral body, above the intervertebral disc (14). Therefore, a small disc prolapse will pass below its own nerve and impinge on the nerve emerging from the next foramen down. For example an L3 prolapse will compress the L4 nerve. More serious disc prolapses extend laterally and may compress the nerve of the same name too.

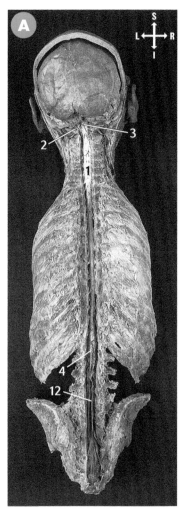

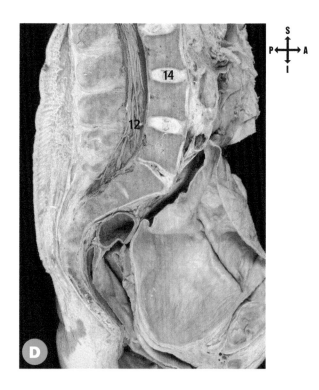

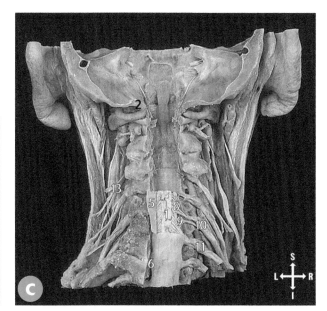

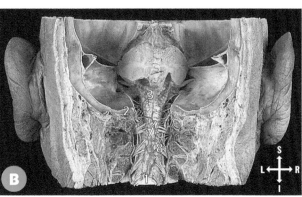

A Skull and vertebral column opened, with spinal cord *in situ* (from behind)

B Brainstem and cervical part of the spinal cord (from behind)

C Vertebral column, cervical region (from behind)

D Pelvis left half in a midline sagittal section (from the right)

1	Spinal cord (spinal medulla)	5	Dura mater (reflected)
2	Margin of foramen magnum	6	Epidural space
3	Medulla oblongata	7	Posterior spinal arteries
4	Lower end of spinal cord	8	Dorsal rootlets of spinal nerve

9	Ventral rootlets of spinal nerve	12	Cauda equina
10	Spinal nerve	13	Ventral rami
11	Dorsal root ganglion within dural sheath	14	Intervertebral disc

Location of numbers: 1ABC; 2ABC; 3AB; 4A; 5C; 6C; 7B; 8BC; 9C; 10C; 11C; 12AD; 13C; 14D.

Part III

Head and Neck

Skull bones and base, external view

The skull bones(1–11) house the brain (surrounded by the meninges and cerebrospinal fluid (CSF)) and the organs of special sense, hearing (plus balance), smell, sight and taste. The nasal and oral cavities are the commencement of the respiratory and gastro-intestinal systems, respectively. The mandible (10) articulates with the skull at the synovial temporomandibular joints (12) for mouth opening and mastication.

From the lateral aspect, the frontal, parietal, temporal (squamous part) and sphenoid (greater wing) meet at the pterion (Illustration C: 'H') in the temporal fossa. The middle meningeal artery has anterior (13) and posterior (14) branches that lie inside the skull and supply the meninges. The anterior branch, deep to the pterion, is particularly vulnerable to external trauma, and rupture causes extradural haemorrhage, i.e. bleeding at arterial pressure between the dura and the overlying bone.

On the skull base, the maxillae house the upper teeth and form much of the hard palate. They also contribute to the face, nasal cavity and orbit. The horizontal plates (15) of the L-shaped palatine bones complete the hard palate. The greater and lesser palatine nerves emerge from foramina in the posterolateral corners. The perpendicular plates (16) contribute to the lateral walls of the nasal cavity.

The body of the sphenoid (17) forms a central strut for the skull base, and gives attachment to the vomer (18), which forms the posterior aspect of the nasal septum. The pterygoid process of the sphenoid divides into medial and lateral plates (19). The medial plate forms the most posterior bony part of the lateral wall of the nasal cavity and gives attachment to the fascia and muscles that form the nasopharynx. The lateral plate gives origin to the pterygoid muscles. The greater wing of the sphenoid is the roof of the infratemporal fossa and has the foramen ovale (20) and, next to its spine, the foramen spinosum (21). The cartilaginous part of the auditory (Eustachian) tube lies in the groove (22) between the greater wing of sphenoid and the petrous temporal bone.

The squamous temporal is seen on the skull base as the mandibular fossa (23) and articular tubercle (24) that form the temporomandibular joint. The tympanic plate is the anterior wall of the external acoustic meatus (25) and the posterior wall of the mandibular fossa. The two bones (squamous and tympanic) fuse at the squamotympanic fissure, which not only gives attachment to the temporomandibular joint capsule, but also has the chorda tympani emerging from its medial end. The styloid process (26) gives origin to muscles that elevate and retract the tongue and pharynx. The mastoid process (27) along with the superior nuchal line is the proximal attachment of sternocleidomastoid and only develops after the infant lifts the head. The petrous temporal bone (28) houses the middle and inner ear. The stylomastoid foramen (29) transmits the facial nerve.

In life the foramen lacerum (30) is filled with cartilage and nothing of importance passes into or out of the skull through it. The internal carotid artery, surrounded by its plexus of sympathetic nerves, passes through the petrous temporal bone in the carotid canal (31), which opens in the skull immediately above the foramen lacerum. The internal jugular vein is formed in the jugular foramen (32), and cranial nerves IX, X and XI emerge from the foramen anterior to the vein.

The occipital bone fuses with the body of the sphenoid anterior to the foramen magnum (33); behind the foramen it forms the posterior aspect of the cranium, which gives attachment to many small but powerful muscles that hold the head extended or rotate it at the atlanto-axial joint. The superior nuchal line (34) gives attachment to trapezius and sternocleidomastoid.

The foramen magnum transmits the medulla to immediately become the spinal cord. All three meninges, the CSF, the spinal roots of the accessory nerve, and the vertebral and spinal arteries pass through the foramen magnum. The occipital condyles (35) form the atlanto-occipital joint for head flexion and extension. The hypoglossal nerve (XII) passes through an anterior canal in the condyle. The large posterior condylar canal (36) transmits an emissary vein.

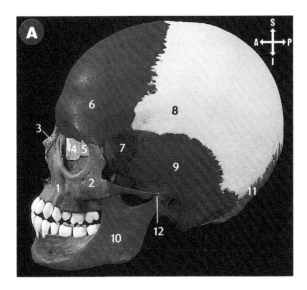

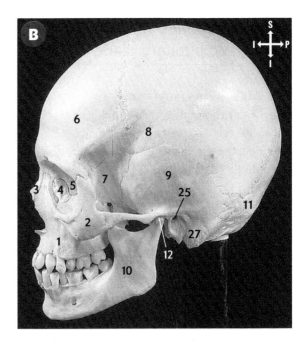

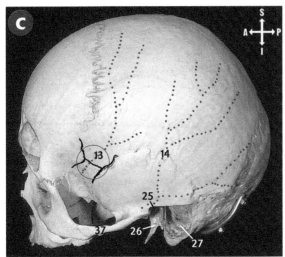

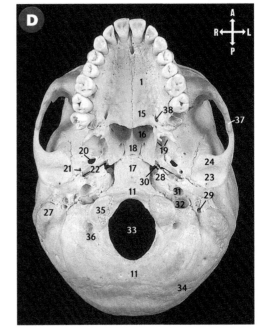

A Skull with individual bones coloured (from the left)

B Skull (from the left)

C Skull without mandible (from the left). 'H' indicates the suture line union of the frontal, parietal, temporal and sphenoid bones. Dotted lines (drill holes) follow the course of grooves on the internal surface of the cranial cavity for branches of the meningeal arteries. The circle indicates the area known as the pterion through the centre of which passes the frontal branch of the middle meningeal artery

D Base of skull, external surface (from below)

1	Maxilla	**12**	Temporomandibular joint	
2	Zygomatic bone	**13**	Position of anterior branch of	
3	Nasal bone		middle meningeal artery	
4	Lacrimal bone	**14**	Position of posterior branch of	
5	Ethmoid bone		middle meningeal artery	
6	Frontal bone	**15**	Horizontal plate of palatine bone	
7	Sphenoid bone	**16**	Perpendicular plate of palatine	
8	Parietal bone		bone	
9	Temporal bone	**17**	Body of sphenoid bone	
10	Mandible	**18**	Vomer	
11	Occipital bone			

19	Medial and lateral pterygoid plates	**28**	Apex of petrous temporal bone
20	Foramen ovale	**29**	Stylomastoid foramen
21	Foramen spinosum	**30**	Foramen lacerum
22	Groove for cartilaginous part of auditory tube	**31**	Carotid canal
23	Mandibular fossa	**32**	Jugular foramen
24	Articular eminence (tubercle)	**33**	Foramen magnum
25	External acoustic meatus	**34**	Superior nuchal line
26	Styloid process	**35**	Occipital condyle
27	Mastoid process	**36**	Posterior condylar canal
		37	Zygomatic arch
		38	Greater palatine foramen

Location of numbers: 1ABD; **2**AB; **3**AB; **4**AB; **5**AB; **6**AB; **7**AB; **8**AB; **9**AB; **10**AB; **11**ABD; **12**AB; **13**C; **14**C; **15**D; **16**D; **17**D; **18**D; **19**D; **20**D; **21**D; **22**D; **23**D; **24**D; **25**BC; **26**C; **27**BCD; **28**D; **29**D; **30**D; **31**D; **32**D; **33**D; **34**D; **35**D; **36**D; **37**CD; **38**D.

Skull bones and base, internal view; pituitary gland

The skull bones (1–11) are seen opposite. The branches of the middle meningeal artery (12,13) are visible in relation to the dura mater (14). When describing the skull base, it is divided into the anterior (A), middle (B) and posterior (C) cranial fossae.

Anterior cranial fossa

The ethmoid bone (11) forms the upper aspect of the nasal cavity and the medial walls of the orbits, which lie on either side of the nasal cavity. The crista galli (17) gives attachment to the falx cerebri. The foramina in the cribriform plate (18) transmit the olfactory nerves. The foramen caecum (19) transmits an emissary vein that may allow spread of infection from outside the skull to inside, which can result in cerebral abscess formation.

As cranial nerves leave the skull they carry with them short extensions of the meninges that cover the brain. Such extensions anchor the olfactory nerves (I) to the cribriform plate. However, the brain and olfactory tracts are able to move within the skull. Consequently, head injury may cause tearing of the olfactory nerves from the olfactory bulb, with resultant loss of the sense of smell (anosmia). Fractures of the cribriform plate may allow cerebrospinal fluid (CSF) to leak into the nose and drip from the nostrils (CSF rhinorrhoea).

The orbital plates (20) of the frontal bone and the lesser wings of the sphenoid (21) form the remainder of the anterior cranial fossa.

Middle cranial fossa

The body (5) and greater wings of the sphenoid (22), with petrous (23) and squamous (6) parts of the temporal bone, form this fossa. The body of the sphenoid extends upward as two posterior clinoid processes. The medial ends of the lesser wings form anterior clinoid processes. The four processes look like a Turkish saddle (sella turcica).

The pituitary gland (hypophysis cerebri) is about the size of a pea and lies under the diaphragma sellae in the pituitary fossa (sella turcica) (24), which places it between the cavernous venous sinuses and above the sphenoid air sinuses. The gland has a posterior neurohypophysis (25) and an anterior adenohypophysis

(26). The former connects to the hypothalamus via the infundibulum and secretes antidiuretic hormone (to control water reabsorption in the kidney) and oxytocin (to control muscle contraction in the uterus and mammary gland). The adenohypophysis secretes many trophic hormones to influence such events as: body growth; adrenal cortical function; thyroid function; cyclical ovarian function; spermatogenesis; pigmentation; and female breast development. A portal circulation that carries releasing factors from the hypothalamus controls hormone release. Tumours of the pituitary gland may be surgically approached via the nasal cavity and sphenoid sinuses.

The optic canal (27) carries the optic nerve (II). The meninges and CSF pass with the nerve to the posterior aspect of the eyeball. Raised intracranial pressure is transmitted along the optic nerve and causes swelling (papilloedema) of the optic disc where the optic nerve enters the eyeball. Such swelling is visible on the retina by ophthalmoscopy.

The superior orbital fissure (28) transmits nerves and vessels to and from the orbit: ophthalmic (V^1), oculomotor (III), trochlear (IV) and abducent (VI) nerves and ophthalmic veins. The foramen spinosum (29) transmits the middle meningeal artery, whereas the foramen ovale (30) transmits the mandibular division of the trigeminal nerve (V^3). The carotid canal opens in the upper aspect of the foramen lacerum (31). Therefore the internal carotid artery lies just to the side of the body of the sphenoid, above the foramen lacerum. A small fossa (32) at the apex of the bone is the site of the trigeminal ganglion.

Posterior cranial fossa

The posterior surface of the petrous temporal bone, the occipital bone, and centrally the clivus (33) (the fused portion of the sphenoid and occipital bones) form the posterior cranial fossa. The overlying dural venous sinuses may indent and mark the bones (34,35).

The internal acoustic meatus (36) transmits the facial (VII) and vestibulocochlear (VIII) nerves. The glossopharyngeal (IX), vagus (X), and accessory (XI) nerves leave the skull through the jugular foramen (37). The foramen magnum (38) transmits the spinal cord, as it becomes the medulla, with its associated meninges and blood vessels.

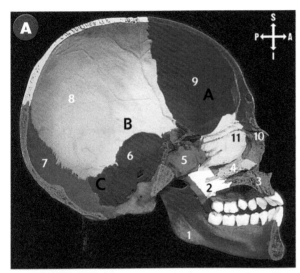

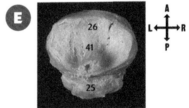

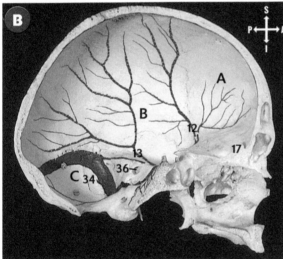

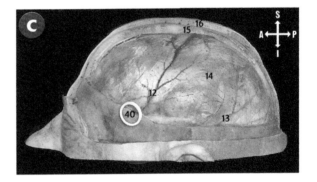

A Left half of skull in a median sagittal section with individual bones coloured. Perpendicular plate of the ethmoid bone removed to expose the superior and middle nasal conchae (from the right)

B Left half of skull in a median sagittal section. Perpendicular plate of the ethmoid bone and mandible removed. Grooves for the meningeal arteries are painted red and sigmoid sinus blue (from the right)

C Dura mater and meningeal vessels (from the left)

D Base of skull, internal surface (from above)

E Pituitary gland (from above)

1 Mandible	**12** Position of anterior branch of middle meningeal artery	**21** Lesser wing of sphenoid bone	**31** Foramen lacerum
2 Palatine bone		**22** Greater wing of sphenoid bone	**32** Trigeminal impression (for ganglion)
3 Maxilla	**13** Position of posterior branch of middle meningeal artery	**23** Petrous temporal bone	
4 Inferior nasal concha		**24** Pituitary fossa (sella turcica)	**33** Clivus
5 Sphenoid bone	**14** Dura mater	**25** Posterior lobe of pituitary gland (neurohypophysis)	**34** Position of sigmoid sinus
6 Squamous part of temporal bone	**15** Bone of cranial vault		**35** Groove for transverse sinus
7 Occipital bone	**16** Scalp	**26** Anterior lobe of pituitary gland (adenohypophysis)	**36** Internal acoustic meatus
8 Parietal bone	**17** Crista galli of ethmoid bone		**37** Jugular foramen
9 Frontal bone	**18** Cribriform plate of ethmoid bone	**27** Optic canal	**38** Foramen magnum
10 Nasal bone		**28** Superior orbital fissure	**39** Internal occipital protuberance
11 Ethmoid bone, superior and middle nasal conchae	**19** Foramen caecum	**29** Foramen spinosum	**40** Position of pterion
	20 Orbital part of frontal bone	**30** Foramen ovale	**41** Pituitary stalk

Location of numbers: 1A; 2A; 3A; 4A; 5AD; 6AD; 7A; 8A; 9A; 10A; 11A; 12BC; 13BC; 14C; 15C; 16C; 17BD; 18D; 19D; 20D; 21D; 22D; 23D; 24D; 25E; 26E; 27D; 28D; 29D; 30D; 31D; 32D; 33D; 34BD; 35D; 36BD; 37D; 38D; 39D; 40C; 41E.

Intracranial view: meninges, sinuses, cerebral veins

Meninges

Inside the skull the brain, like the spinal cord, is surrounded by the three meninges. The thin, hardly visible membrane of pia mater (1) clothes the brain. The arachnoid mater (2) covers the brain but does not dip into the fissures and sulci. It more closely follows the contours of the overlying dura mater (3) and skull.

Cerebrospinal fluid (CSF) fills the space between the pia and the arachnoid, providing a buoyant waterbed upon which the brain is cushioned. The CSF is continually synthesized by choroid plexus within the ventricles of the brain and flows into the subarachnoid space. The amount of CSF is normally 120–150 mL. It is reabsorbed via arachnoid villi that cluster in granulations (4) that push into the venous sinuses of the dura mater.

Within the skull the dura mater is described as having a meningeal and a periosteal layer. The two are fused together except at specific sites. The periosteal layer is adherent to the inner surface of the skull and is continuous with the fibrous tissue of the sutures between the skull bones. At the foramina, the periosteal layer of dura is continuous with the periosteum external to the skull. The meningeal layer separates from the periosteal layer to leave endothelially-lined dural venous sinuses in the resultant spaces. The meningeal layer also separates to form two double folds of dura mater, the falx cerebri (5) and tentorium cerebelli (6).

The falx cerebri passes from the crista galli to the internal occipital protuberance (7). It separates the cerebral hemispheres (8), preventing their shifting during rotational movements of the head. Head injury may force the brain sharply against the firm falx causing cerebral contusion.

The tentorium cerebelli, as the name suggests forms a roof over the cerebellum (9) separating it from the occipital lobe (10) of the brain. Its attached margin encloses the transverse sinuses (11) and the superior petrosal sinuses (12) on the posterosuperior edges of the petrous temporal bones. Its free margin (13) forms the tentorial notch, through which the brain stem (14) passes. Lesions in the posterior cranial fossa are infratentorial, those above are supratentorial.

Dural venous sinuses

The superior sagittal sinus (15) is in the attached margin of the falx. It usually continues as the right transverse sinus. The inferior sagittal sinus, in the free (inferior) margin of the falx (16) usually enters the straight sinus (17) in the junction between the falx cerebri and the tentorium cerebelli. The straight sinus usually continues as the left transverse sinus. The straight, superior sagittal and both transverse sinuses may all join at the confluence of the sinuses deep to the internal occipital protuberance. From the protuberance the right and left transverse sinuses pass laterally to become the right and left (18) sigmoid sinuses. The inferior petrosal sinuses lie between the clivus and the apices of the petrous temporal bone. Each sigmoid sinus becomes the internal jugular vein in the jugular foramen, and here the inferior petrosal sinus joins the vein.

A cavernous sinus lies on each side of the body of the sphenoid and pituitary gland (19). Each one extends from the apex of the petrous temporal bone anteriorly toward the superior orbital fissure and foramen rotundum. The internal carotid artery emerges from the carotid canal and bends to pass anteriorly within the cavernous sinus. It then curves back upon itself. The series of bends is the carotid siphon that is said to reduce the pressure of blood flow within the artery. Rarely, an arteriovenous fistula may form between the artery and the sinus.

Cerebral veins drain the deep parts of the brain and converge on the great cerebral vein that enters the straight sinus. More superficially, cerebral veins cross the subarachnoid space to enter the venous sinuses, particularly the superior sagittal sinus.

The brain shrinks slightly with age, causing mild traction on these cerebral veins. Relatively minor trauma may damage the veins just as they enter the sinus, causing subdural venous haemorrhage.

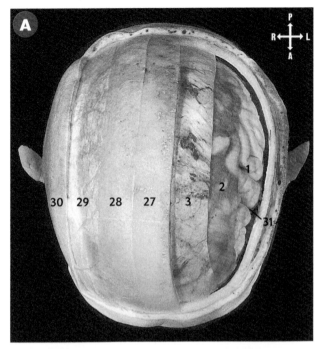

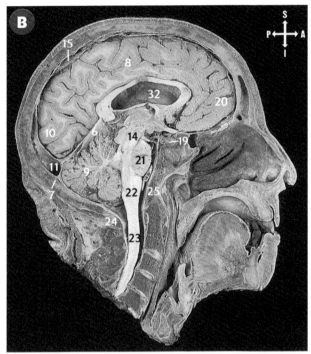

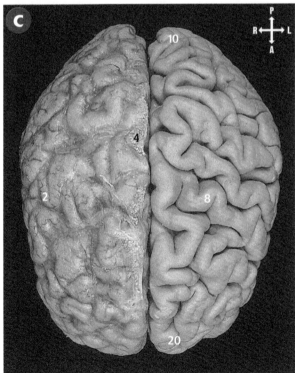

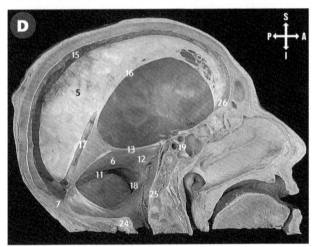

A Stepped dissection of scalp and cranial vault (from above)
B Cranial cavity and brain in a median sagittal section (from the right)
C Brain, cerebral hemispheres (from above)
D Cranial cavity in median sagittal section (from the right)

1	Cerebral hemisphere covered by pia mater	**10**	Occipital lobe (pole)
2	Arachnoid mater	**11**	Transverse sinus
3	Dura mater	**12**	Position of superior petrosal sinus
4	Arachnoid granulations	**13**	Free margin of tentorium cerebelli
5	Falx cerebri	**14**	Brain stem
6	Tentorium cerebelli	**15**	Superior sagittal sinus
7	Internal occipital protuberance	**16**	Inferior margin of falx cerebri
8	Cerebral hemisphere	**17**	Straight sinus
9	Cerebellum		

18	Sigmoid sinus	**26**	Crista galli of ethmoid bone
19	Pituitary gland	**27**	Bone of cranial vault
20	Frontal lobe (pole)	**28**	Loose connective tissue and pericranium
21	Pons	**29**	Epicranial aponeurosis (galea aponeurotica)
22	Medulla oblongata	**30**	Skin and dense subcutaneous tissue
23	Spinal cord (spinal medulla)	**31**	Subarachnoid space
24	Posterior margin of foramen magnum	**32**	Lateral ventricle
25	Anterior margin of foramen magnum		

Location of numbers: 1A; **2**AC; **3**A; **4**C; **5**D; **6**BD; **7**BD; **8**BC; **9**B; **10**BC; **11**BD; **12**D; **13**D; **14**B; **15**BD; **16**D; **17**D; **18**D; **19**BD; **20**BC; **21**B; **22**B; **23**B; **24**BD; **25**BD; **26**D; **27**A; **28**A; **29**A; **30**A; **31**A; **32**B.

Brain, cerebral arteries

The soft, live brain is supported by the three meninges, pia, arachnoid (1) and dura mater, as well as the cerebrospinal fluid (CSF) in the subarachnoid space. The brain is divided into left and right hemispheres. Each has a ventricle (2) that extends from the parietal (3) into the frontal (4), occipital (5) and temporal (6) lobes. These lateral ventricles communicate with the third ventricle (7) that lies between the two hemispheres. The third ventricle leads to the fourth via the narrow cerebral aqueduct (8). Vascular choroid plexuses produce CSF, which is exported via foramina in the fourth ventricle (9) to fill the sub-arachnoid space. In the newborn, obstruction of the normal flow of CSF causes hydrocephaly.

The frontal lobe, anterior to the central sulcus (12), controls the execution and direction of motor function, as well as personality and judgement. Broca's area (13) controls speech, and the frontal eye field (14) controls eye movement. The parietal lobe is for the reception, recognition and memory of general sensation. The occipital lobe, around the calcarine sulcus (15), has these functions for vision. The temporal lobe is associated with hearing and emotion. The two hemispheres communicate with each other via the corpus callosum (16).

Motor principles

Nerve fibres or upper motor neurones (UMNs) descend, mainly from the precentral gyrus (17), through the internal capsule to the medulla (18), where they usually cross the midline before impinging on clusters of cells in the anterior horn of the spinal cord. These cells, or lower motor neurones (LMNs) send axons to muscles in the periphery. Cortical control is inverted (upper brain/lower body) as well as crossed (left hemisphere/right side of body). Upper motor neurones have excitatory and inhibitory effects on the LMNs. Damage to the UMN classically causes weakness, spasticity, increased reflexes and up-going toes.

Descending cortical fibres also project to the basal ganglia and, via the pons (19), to the cerebellum (20). The latter receives ascending, proprioceptive input from the muscles and joints of the body. The basal ganglia and cerebellum create circuits to memorize, direct and co-ordinate motor function.

Cranial nerve nuclei in the brain stem usually receive descending cortical fibres bilaterally. But cortical supply to the nucleus of the facial nerve is important. The upper part of the nucleus receives supply from both the left and right cortices, i.e. bilateral supply. The lower part of the nucleus receives supply only from the opposite cortex. Therefore, a cerebrovascular 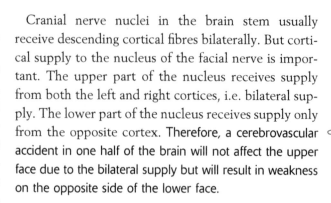accident in one half of the brain will not affect the upper face due to the bilateral supply but will result in weakness on the opposite side of the lower face.

Sensory principles

The cell bodies of sensory neurones are clustered in ganglia lying just outside the central nervous system. The central processes enter the spinal cord, and synapse with the secondary neurones either immediately (pain and temperature) or in the medulla (discriminative touch and proprioception). The secondary neurones cross the midline and ascend to the thalamus from where the tertiary neurones go to the postcentral gyrus (21) of the cortex. Representation is crossed and inverted. Cranial nerves usually project bilaterally. All sensation reaches the cortex via the thalamus.

Spinal or brain stem reflex arcs link the sensory input to the motor output via interneurones.

Arteries

The internal carotid artery (22) emerges from the petrous temporal bone and bends to pass anteriorly within the cavernous sinus. It then curves back upon itself, gives off its first branch, the ophthalmic artery and divides into the middle (23) and anterior (24) cerebral arteries.

The left and right vertebral arteries (25) fuse to form the basilar artery (26). They supply the spinal cord, the cerebellum and pons. The basilar artery divides into the posterior cerebral arteries (27). Posterior communicating arteries (28) pass from the posterior cerebrals to the middle cerebrals and the anterior communicating artery (29) links the two anterior cerebrals. This arrangement creates the anastomotic arterial Circle (of Willis) (Illustration D) to supply the brain. The arteries lie within the CSF. Small aneurysms may form as the arteries bifurcate; these are prone to rupture causing subarachnoid haemorrhage.

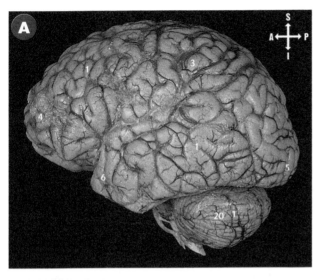

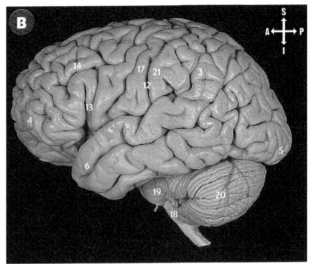

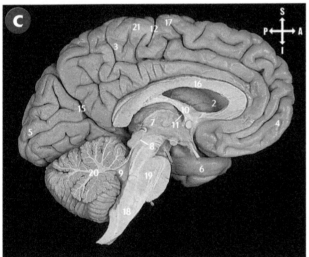

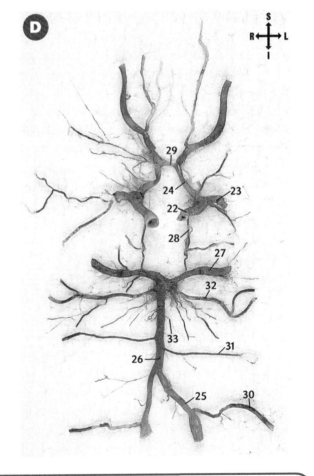

A Brain, external, veins (from the left)
B Brain, external, sulci (from the left)
C Brain and brainstem, left half (from the right)
D Arterial circle (of Willis) and associated vessels of the base of brain (from below)

1	Arachnoid mater	9	Fourth ventricle	18	Medulla oblongata	27	Posterior cerebral artery
2	Lateral ventricle	10	Body of fornix	19	Pons	28	Posterior communicating artery
3	Parietal lobe (pole)	11	Interventricular foramen	20	Cerebellum	29	Anterior communicating artery
4	Frontal lobe (pole)	12	Central sulcus	21	Postcentral gyrus	30	Posterior inferior cerebellar
5	Occipital lobe (pole)	13	Broca's speech area	22	Internal carotid artery		artery
6	Temporal lobe (pole)	14	Left frontal eye field	23	Middle cerebral artery	31	Anterior inferior cerebellar artery
7	Thalamus lateral to third	15	Calcarine sulcus	24	Anterior cerebral artery	32	Superior cerebellar artery
	ventricle	16	Corpus callosum	25	Vertebral artery	33	Labyrinthine artery
8	Aqueduct of midbrain	17	Precentral gyrus	26	Basilar artery		

Location of numbers: 1A; 2C; 3ABC; 4ABC; 5ABC; 6ABC; 7C; 8C; 9C; 10C; 11C; 12BC; 13B 14B; 15C; 16C; 17BC; 18BC; 19BC; 20ABC; 21BC; 22D; 23D; 24D; 25D; 26D; 27D; 28D; 29D; 30D; 31D; 32D; 33D.

Intracranial view: introduction to cranial nerves

Twelve pairs of cranial nerves emerge from the brain or brainstem and exit the skull.

Olfactory nerve (I) is for the sense of smell and arises from the olfactory bulb (1) at the distal end of the olfactory tract (2). Optic nerve (II) (3) is for the sense of sight. The nerves converge at the optic chiasma (4) just above and in front of the pituitary gland (5). Tumours of the gland may extend upward and impinge upon the chiasma to cause bitemporal hemianopia.

Oculomotor nerve (III) (6) supplies all but two of the muscles that move the eye, and carries parasympathetic fibres to constrict the pupil. It arises from the brain stem just anterior to the pons (7) and lies on the edge of the tentorium cerebelli (8). Lesions such as abscesses, tumours and haemorrhages may raise the intracranial pressure and force the brain and brain stem inferiorly (coning). The oculomotor nerve may be compressed and damaged against the edge of the tentorium, with resultant eye signs. In an acute episode, the patient will be losing consciousness, or be unconscious, and the important sign is failure of the pupil to constrict to light. Trochlear nerve (IV) (9) supplies the superior oblique muscle. It is a thin nerve that emerges from the posterior aspect of the brain stem and lies in the free edge of the tentorium.

Trigeminal nerve (V) (10) passes anteriorly to reach its ganglion (11) in an invagination of dura mater just under the posterior end of the cavernous sinus. It has three divisions, ophthalmic (V^1) (12), maxillary (V^2) (13) and mandibular (V^3) (14). It is the sensory nerve of much of the head, face and orbital, nasal and oral cavities. The ganglion contains the cell bodies of the primary sensory neurones. The motor root supplies the muscles of mastication via V^3.

Abducent nerve (VI) (16) arises immediately caudal to the pons and passes upward on the clivus. The upward course makes it particularly susceptible to any downward traction on the brain created by raised intracranial pressure. There is resultant paralysis of lateral rectus

and the affected eye cannot be abducted. Nerves III, IV, V^1 and V^2 lie in the lateral wall of the cavernous sinus, and VI lies in the sinus.

Facial nerve (VII) (17) is the motor supply to the muscles of facial expression. It passes through the middle ear and emerges from the stylomastoid foramen. The facial nerve carries with it (nervus intermedius) parasympathetic fibres that leave in the greater petrosal nerve and the chorda tympani, as well as fibres for the sensation of taste. The greater petrosal is secretomotor to the lacrimal, nasal and palatine glands. Its nerve fibres synapse in the pterygopalatine (hay fever) ganglion. Postganglionic fibres are distributed with branches of V^2. The chorda tympani carries taste from the anterior two-thirds of the tongue and is also secretomotor to the submandibular and sublingual salivary glands. It joins the lingual branch of V^3, and its parasympathetic fibres synapse in the submandibular ganglion. Its taste fibres have their cell bodies in the geniculate ganglion, visible as a swelling on the facial nerve in the middle ear.

Vestibulocochlear (VIII) (18) supplies the organs responsible for hearing and balance. Glossopharyngeal (IX) (19) supplies one muscle (stylopharyngeus) and carries general sensation and taste from the posterior one-third of the tongue, the oropharynx and the palatine tonsil. It also carries parasympathetic fibres that run with its tympanic branch, which supplies sensation to the middle ear.

Vagus (X) (20) supplies the musculature of the pharynx and larynx, and is the parasympathetic nerve to the heart, lungs and much of the intestinal tract. Ganglionic swellings on the vagus house the cell bodies of the afferent nerves from the pharynx, larynx, heart, lungs and intestine. Accessory (XI) (21) is actually a spinal nerve arising from C1–5 segments of the spinal cord. It ascends up the spinal canal and through the foramen magnum to pass through the jugular foramen to supply sternocleidomastoid and trapezius. Hypoglossal nerve (XII) is a totally motor nerve to the tongue muscles. It is at risk of injury during carotid artery surgery in the neck.

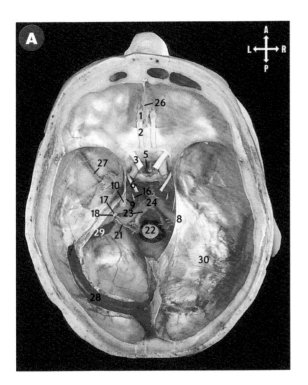

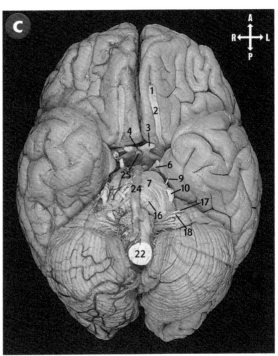

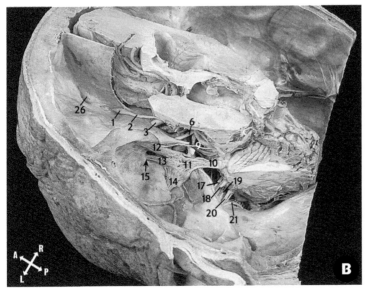

A Cranial fossae (from above)
B Cranial fossae, left cavernous sinus and
   trigeminal nerve (from above and left)
C Brain and brainstem (from below)

1 Olfactory bulb	**9** Trochlear nerve (IV)	**18** Vestibulocochlear nerve (VIII)	**26** Falx cerebri attached to crista
2 Olfactory tract	**10** Trigeminal nerve (V)	**19** Glossopharyngeal nerve (IX)	galli of ethmoid bone
3 Optic nerve (II)	**11** Trigeminal ganglion	**20** Vagus nerve (X)	**27** Middle meningeal artery
4 Optic chiasma	**12** Ophthalmic nerve (V¹)	**21** Spinal root of accessory nerve	**28** Transverse sinus
5 Pituitary gland	**13** Maxillary nerve (V²)	(XI)	**29** Sigmoid sinus
6 Oculomotor nerve (III)	**14** Mandibular nerve (V³)	**22** Medulla oblongata	**30** Tentorium cerebelli
7 Pons	**15** Foramen rotundum	**23** Vertebral artery	
8 Free margin of tentorium	**16** Abducent nerve (VI)	**24** Basilar artery	
cerebelli	**17** Facial nerve (VII)	**25** Pituitary stalk	

Location of numbers: 1ABC; **2**ABC; **3**ABC; **4**C; **5**A; **6**ABC; **7**C; **8**A; **9**ABC; **10**ABC; **11**B; **12**B; **13**B; **14**B; **15**B; **16**AC; **17**ABC; **18**ABC; **19**B; **20**B; **21**AB; **22**AC; **23**A; **24**AC; **25**C; **26**AB; **27**A; **28**A; **29**A; **30**A.

Ear, associated nerves

The ear, for hearing and balance, comprises the auricle (pinna), external acoustic meatus (1), tympanic membrane (2), middle ear and inner ear. Much of the ear is housed within the temporal bone and is closely related to the sigmoid venous sinus, middle cranial fossa and internal carotid artery.

The auricle (3–10) (Illustration C), supported by elastic cartilage (Illustration B), gathers sound. Small, rarely used extrinsic muscles (supplied by VII) insert into the auricle to move it and minimally alter its shape. The external acoustic meatus has a cartilaginous lateral third and a bony medial two-thirds. It is S-shaped and about 2.5 cm long in the adult, but shorter in the infant. The skin is firmly bound to the underlying bone and cartilage and therefore, inflammation is painful. Ceruminous glands (modified sweat glands) secrete wax, which may block the meatus. When using an auriscope, gently drawing the auricle upward and backward tends to straighten the meatus.

The tympanic membrane is oval in shape, slopes inferomedially, and bulges inward toward the middle ear, the umbo being the point of maximal convexity. There is an upper, flaccid part, but the remainder is tense. The malleus attaches to its inner surface.

The middle ear is like a biconcave lens. It is filled with air and houses the malleus, incus and stapes, which transmit sound waves from the tympanic membrane to the cochlea. Tensor tympani (V^3) and stapedius (VII) attach to these ossicles to dampen excessive vibration. The auditory tube (middle ear to nasopharynx) equalizes air pressure on either side of the tympanic membrane. Patency of the tube is essential for normal ear function. The epitympanic recess is the upper aspect of the middle ear and connects via the mastoid antrum (17) to the mastoid air cells in the mastoid process (18). Middle ear infection may spread to the air cells (mastoiditis).

The inner ear houses the bony labyrinth, itself lined by the fluid-filled membranous labyrinth, and subdivided into the cochlea (hearing) and semicircular canals with utricle and saccule (balance). The stapes attaches to the oval window of the cochlea to transmit sound waves via the organ of Corti to the cochlear nerve. The semicircular canals are angled to each other and detect head position for balance, transmitted in the vestibular nerve.

The internal acoustic meatus (19) transmits VII and VIII with the labyrinthine branch of the basilar artery. Tumours (e.g. acoustic neuromas) may expand into the internal acoustic meatus and into the angle between the pons and cerebellum to impinge upon these nerves.

Nerves

The auriculotemporal nerve (V^3 (20)) is the main sensory supply of the auricle, external acoustic meatus and external aspect of the tympanic membrane. The latter two are also supplied by the vagus, – thought to carry a sensory branch of the facial nerve. Herpes affecting the geniculate ganglion (21) (VII) may affect the external meatus (Ramsay–Hunt syndrome) and ear examination may affect heart rate via the vagus. The great auricular and lesser occipital nerves also supply the auricle.

Middle ear sensation (and that of the internal aspect of the tympanic membrane) is via the tympanic branch of the glossopharyngeal nerve, which also carries parasympathetic (secretomotor) nerves to the tympanic plexus in the middle ear. These leave in the lesser petrosal nerve, which synapses in the otic ganglion suspended from V^3 just below the foramen ovale. Postganglionic fibres pass in the auriculotemporal nerve to the parotid gland.

The facial nerve gives a number of branches as it passes through the middle ear. It supplies the stapedius muscle, and proximal injury to the facial nerve will cause hyperacusis (pain on loud noises). The chorda tympani arises from it and passes medial to the tympanic membrane. The greater petrosal nerve (26) arises from the geniculate ganglion and passes to synapse in the pterygopalatine ganglion in the pterygopalatine fossa. The fossa is medial to the pterygomaxillary fissure (27), lateral to the nasal cavity and nasopharynx, posterior to the orbit and inferior orbital fissure, and superior to the hard and soft palates. The maxillary nerve V^2 (28) enters the fossa via the foramen rotundum.

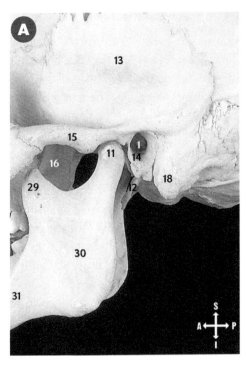

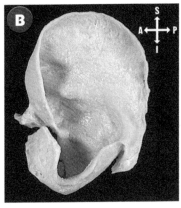

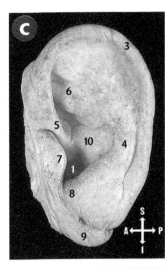

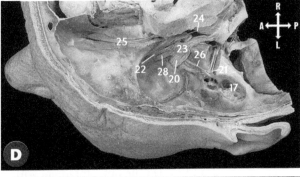

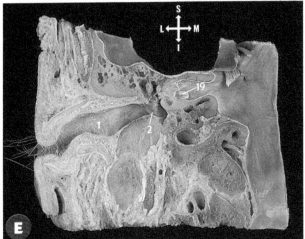

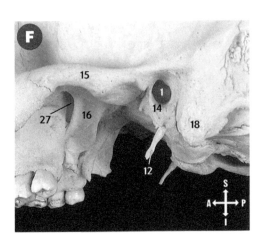

A Skull and mandible (from the left)
B Left auricular cartilage (from the left)
C Left auricle (from the left)
D Cranial fossae, temporal bone dissected to expose the auditory ossicles (from above and left)
E Coronal section through the left ear (from behind)
F Skull without mandible (from the left and slightly below)

1	External acoustic meatus	**10**	Cavum conchae	**17**	Mastoid antrum	**24** Trochlear nerve (IV)
2	Tympanic membrane	**11**	Head of mandible	**18**	Mastoid process	**25** Olfactory tract
3	Helix	**12**	Styloid process	**19**	Facial nerve (VII) and	**26** Greater petrosal nerve
4	Antihelix	**13**	Squamous part of temporal		vestibulocochlear nerve (VIII)	**27** Pterygomaxillary fissure
5	Crus of helix		bone		within the internal acoustic meatus	**28** Maxillary nerve (V²)
6	Crus of antihelix	**14**	Tympanic plate of temporal bone	**20**	Mandibular nerve (V³)	**29** Coronoid process of mandible
7	Tragus	**15**	Zygomatic arch	**21**	Geniculate ganglion	**30** Ramus of mandible
8	Antitragus	**16**	Lateral pterygoid plate of	**22**	Ophthalmic nerve (V¹)	**31** Body of mandible
9	Lobule		sphenoid bone	**23**	Trigeminal ganglion	

Location of numbers: **1**ACEF; **2**E; **3**C; **4**C; **5**C; **6**C; **7**C; **8**C; **9**C; **10**C; **11**A; **12**AF; **13**A; **14**AF; **15**AF; **16**AF; **17**D; **18**AF; **19**E; **20**D; **21**D; **22**D; **23**D; **24**D; **25**D; **26**D; **27**F; **28**D; **29**A; **30**A; **31**A.

Orbital skeleton, eyelids, conjunctiva

The eyeballs are surrounded by muscles and supported by fat within the orbit. They must maintain their position and move in absolute synchrony, or double vision (diplopia) will ensue.

Each bony orbit opens on the facial skull, bounded by the frontal bone (1), zygomatic bone (2) and maxilla (3). The orbit is cone-shaped with the apex passing backward and medially. This angulation is important when considering the actions of the orbital muscles.

Orbital skeleton, foramina, fissures and their contents

- Medial wall – mainly by the lacrimal (4) and ethmoid (5) bones.
- Roof – the orbital part (6) of the frontal and lesser wing of the sphenoid bone (7). The optic foramen or canal (8) is at the apex of the orbit, in the roots of the lesser wing of the sphenoid. The optic nerve enters the orbit through the optic foramen, with the ophthalmic branch of the internal carotid artery. The central artery of the retina arises from the ophthalmic and passes into the optic nerve to supply both it and the retina. Being an end artery, obstruction of the central artery leads to blindness in that eye.
- Lateral wall – greater wing of sphenoid (9) and zygomatic bone. The superior orbital fissure (10) is between the roof and lateral wall, i.e. between the lesser and greater wings of the sphenoid.
- Floor – maxilla. The inferior orbital fissure (11) is between the lateral wall and the floor, i.e. between the greater wing of the sphenoid and the maxilla. The maxillary (V²) division of the trigeminal nerve continues through the inferior orbital fissure as the infra-orbital nerve, which runs in the infra-orbital groove (12) in the orbital floor. (The infra-orbital groove in some skulls is closed and then named the infra-orbital canal.) The nerve emerges from the infra-orbital foramen (13) to supply the skin and conjunctiva of the lower eyelid, cheek and upper lip.

Eyelids and lacrimal mechanism

The skin of the eyelids is thin with no subcutaneous fat. The eyelashes (14) line the edge of each lid to prevent dust entering the eye. Like all hairs they have sebaceous glands alongside. These may become infected and form a 'sty'. Orbicularis oculi underlies the skin. It has an orbital part (15) that encircles the orbit to screw the eyes tightly shut, and a palpebral part (16) in the eyelids for blinking and keeping the eyelids opposed to the eyeball. The latter action is essential for correct function of the lacrimal mechanism; should the muscle or its nerve supply (VII) be injured the lid may fall away from the eye. Tears will then run down the face, possibly leaving the cornea dry and susceptible to ulceration.

Tarsal plates of fibrous tissue lie deep to orbicularis oculi to give a stiffening support to each lid. Medial and lateral palpebral ligaments connect them to the orbital margins. Meibomian glands lie in the deep surface of the tarsal plates. These secrete an oily fluid to prevent evaporation and keep the eye moist. Cysts may form in the Meibomian glands. The conjunctival membrane lines the inner aspect of both lids. It is continuous with the skin at the free margins of the lids, but internally it reflects onto the front of the eyeball to become continuous with the corneal epithelium.

The lacrimal gland (Illustrations D, E, F (17)) lies in the upper, lateral corner of the orbit and secretes into the conjunctival sac. Blinking of the eyelids sweeps the tears across the eye from lateral to medial to moisten and cleanse the eye. There is a punctum medially in each lid to collect tears, pass them to the lacrimal sac (18) and then, via the nasolacrimal duct (19), to the nose. Part of orbicularis oculi encircles the lacrimal sac to promote the flow of tears into the lacrimal sac and from there into the nasolacrimal duct, obstruction of which causes tears to flow onto the face.

The sensory supply of the cornea, conjunctiva and eyelids is by branches of V¹ and V² (trigeminal nerve). The corneal reflex, blinking when the cornea is touched, is via the nasociliary branch of the ophthalmic (sensory) and facial (motor) nerves.

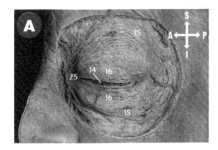

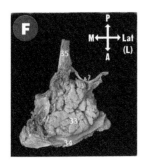

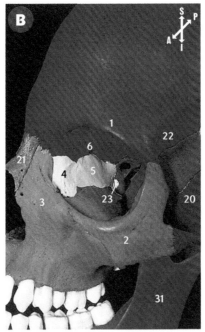

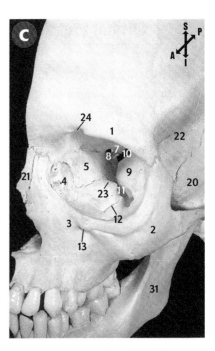

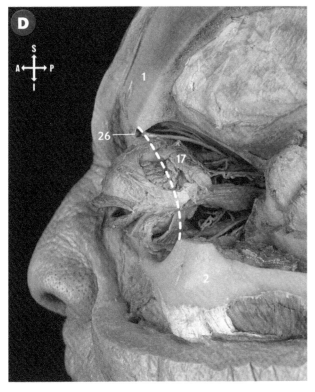

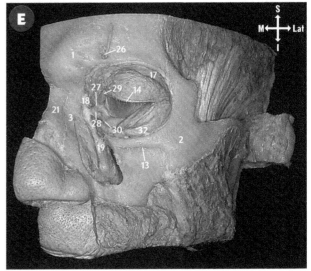

A Superficial muscles of the eye (from the front left)
B Orbit with individual bones coloured (from the front left and above)
C Orbit (from the front and left)
D Orbit (from the front left and above)
E Nasolacrimal duct (from the front and left)
F Left lacrimal gland (from above)

1	Frontal bone	10	Superior orbital fissure
2	Zygomatic bone	11	Inferior orbital fissure
3	Maxilla	12	Infra-orbital groove (canal)
4	Lacrimal bone	13	Infra-orbital foramen
5	Ethmoid bone	14	Eyelashes of upper lid
6	Orbital part of frontal bone	15	Orbital part of orbicularis oculi
7	Lesser wing of sphenoid bone	16	Palpebral part of orbicularis oculi
8	Optic canal	17	Lacrimal gland
9	Greater wing of sphenoid bone orbital aspect	18	Lacrimal sac (upper extremity)
		19	Nasolacrimal duct

20	Temporal bone	29	Upper lacrimal papilla and punctum
21	Nasal bone		
22	Greater wing of sphenoid bone (external aspect)	30	Lower lacrimal papilla and punctum
23	Palatine bone (orbital part)	31	Mandible
24	Supra-orbital foramen (notch)	32	Orbital fat pad
25	Medial palpebral ligament	33	Orbital part of lacrimal gland
26	Supra-orbital artery and nerve	34	Palpebral part of lacrimal gland
27	Upper lacrimal canaliculus	35	Lacrimal artery and nerve
28	Lower lacrimal canaliculus		

Location of numbers: **1**BCDE; **2**BCDE; **3**BCE; **4**BC; **5**BC; **6**B; **7**C; **8**C; **9**C; **10**C; **11**C; **12**C; **13**CE; **14**AE; **15**A; **16**A; **17**DEF; **18**E; **19**E; **20**BC; **21**BCE; **22**BC; **23**BC; **24**C; **25**A; **26**DE; **27**E; **28**E; **29**E; **30**E; **31**BC; **32**E; **33**F; **34**F; **35**F.

Orbital muscles, nerves

There are six muscles for moving the eyeball and one for elevating the upper lid.

Levator palpebrae superioris (3) arises from the orbital roof and passes to the tarsal plate in the upper lid. It contains smooth and striated muscle, supplied by the oculomotor nerve (III) (4) and by sympathetics. Both are required to hold up the upper eyelid. If either is lost, the lid droops (ptosis).

Four rectus muscles (6–9) arise from a tendinous ring encircling the optic foramen and medial end of the superior orbital fissure, so many orbital nerves lie within the cone of these four muscles as they pass forward and laterally to insert near the front of the eyeball. Superior rectus (III) turns the eye upward. Medial rectus (III) turns the eye medially. Inferior rectus (III) turns the eye downward. Lateral rectus (VI) turns the eye laterally. As the origin of superior and inferior recti is posteromedial to the eyeball they impart a medial pull.

Superior oblique (10) (IV) arises above the tendinous ring. It passes forward and through a fibrous trochlea or pulley (11) before turning backward and laterally to insert on the posterolateral aspect of the eyeball. It turns the eye down and out. Inferior oblique (12) (III) arises from the orbital floor and passes to the posterolateral aspect of the eyeball. It turns the eye up and out.

Working in concert the muscles have the following actions:

- Look up – Superior rectus, inferior oblique.
- Look down – Inferior rectus, superior oblique.
- Look medially – Medial rectus, superior and inferior rectus.
- Look laterally – Lateral rectus, inferior and superior oblique.

The muscles also rotate the eyeball to counteract tilting of the head.

Nerves within the orbit

Branches of the ophthalmic (V^1): the lacrimal nerve (13) supplies the upper lateral lid, conjunctiva and adjacent area. It receives parasympathetic fibres for secretomotor control of the lacrimal gland. The frontal nerve lies just beneath the roof of the orbit. It divides into supra-orbital (15) and supratrochlear (16) nerve, which supply skin and conjunctiva of the upper lid, forehead, and scalp to the vertex. The nasociliary nerve (17), as well as being sensory, carries sympathetic fibres from the carotid plexus. These joined the oculomotor nerve in the cavernous sinus. Its ethmoidal branches supply the ethmoidal sinuses (18). The anterior ethmoidal nerve continues into the nasal cavity to supply the anterior aspects of the lateral wall and septum, before emerging to supply the skin of the tip of the nose.

The nasociliary nerve ends as the small infratrochlear nerve, supplying sensation to skin and conjunctiva at the medial angle of the eye, and the root of the nose. Sympathetic and sensory fibres leave the nasociliary in the long ciliary nerves to enter the posterior aspect of the eyeball. The sympathetic fibres are postganglionic, from the superior cervical ganglion, and are for dilatation of the pupil. The sensory fibres supply all the fascial layers of the eyeball including the cornea.

The oculomotor nerve (III) carries parasympathetic fibres that synapse in the ciliary ganglion (19). The postganglionic fibres pass in the short ciliary nerves into the eyeball to the constrictor of the pupil and to ciliaris muscle for lens accommodation. Oculomotor nerve injury causes: pupil dilatation (sympathetic takes over); ptosis (loss of levator palpebrae superioris); and the eye drifts down and out under the control of lateral rectus and superior oblique. There is double vision (diplopia) on looking medially. Damage to sympathetic fibres (Horner's syndrome) also causes ptosis, but with a constricted pupil. The face is flushed and the skin dry on the affected side.

Abducent nerve (VI) (20) injury prevents the eye moving laterally. Trochlear nerve (IV) (21) injury prevents the action of superior oblique. One would expect difficulty looking down and out. However, lateral rectus and inferior rectus perform that function. The test is to ask the patient to look downward and inward. When the eye is turned medially by medial rectus, inferior rectus cannot act effectively, leaving superior oblique as the only muscle to turn the eye downward. If its action is absent the patient cannot do so and has difficulty walking downstairs or looking downward to read.

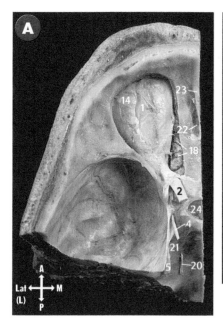

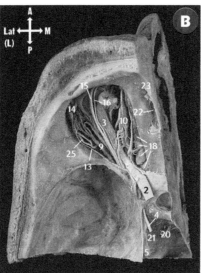

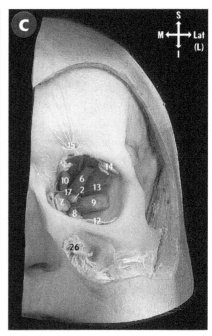

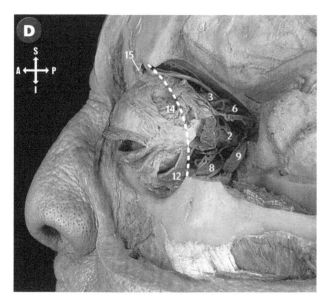

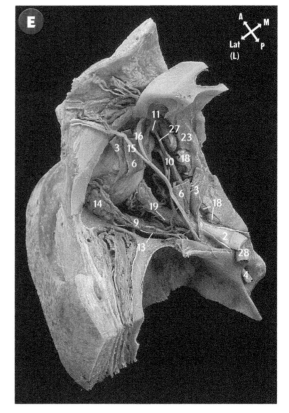

A Orbit with roof removed (from above and behind)
B Orbit, superficial dissection (from above and behind)
C Orbit with eye removed (from the front)
D Orbit, contents with extensive bone removal (from the left)
E Orbit, contents with extensive bone removal (from above left and behind)

1	Orbital fat	9	Lateral rectus
2	Optic nerve (II)	10	Superior oblique
3	Levator palpebrae superioris	11	Trochlea
4	Oculomotor nerve (III)	12	Inferior oblique
5	Trigeminal nerve (V)	13	Lacrimal nerve
6	Superior rectus	14	Lacrimal gland
7	Medial rectus	15	Supra-orbital nerve
8	Inferior rectus	16	Supratrochlear nerve

17	Nasociliary nerve	24	Pituitary gland
18	Ethmoidal air cells	25	Lacrimal artery
19	Ciliary ganglion	26	Infra-orbital nerve
20	Abducent nerve (VI)	27	Tendon of superior oblique
21	Trochlear nerve (IV)	28	Internal carotid artery
22	Cribriform plate of ethmoid bone		
23	Crista galli of ethmoid bone		

Location of numbers: **1**A; **2**ABCDE; **3**BDE; **4**ABE; **5**AB; **6**CDE; **7**C; **8**CD; **9**BCDE; **10**BCE; **11**E; **12**CD; **13**BCE; **14**ABCDE; **15**BCDE; **16**BE; **17**C; **18**ABE; **19**E; **20**AB; **21**AB; **22**AB; **23**ABE; **24**A; **25**B; **26**C; **27**E; **28**E.

Nasal cavity, bones, sinuses, conchae and meati

The nasal cavity is for the sense of smell, and to filter, warm and humidify inhaled air. The highly vascular mucous membrane is firmly attached to the underlying periosteum and contains mucous glands (mucoperiosteum). The overlying epithelium is ciliated, pseudostratified columnar with mucus-secreting goblet cells. The cilia and mucus trap and filter particles, the mucus humidifies, and the vascularity of the mucosa warms the inspired air. Coarse hairs (1), the first filters, are obvious in the nostrils.

The variable diameter of the passages ensures efficient airflow. To withstand the collapsing effect of inspiratory pressure, the nasal cavity is supported by bone and hyaline cartilages. The nasal bones (2) and nasal cartilages (3, 4) shape the visible nose. The small muscles around the nostrils are for their constriction and dilatation, to decrease respiratory dead space, or widen the nostrils for faster air flow.

The midline septum (5) is formed by the vomer (6), the perpendicular plate of the ethmoid (7), and the septal cartilage (8). A deviated septum may obstruct sinus openings, predisposing to sinusitis. Each lateral wall is formed from anterior to posterior by the nasal, maxillary, lacrimal, ethmoid, and palatine bones, and the medial pterygoid plate of sphenoid. The major contributors are maxilla, for the lower half, and ethmoid, for the upper half.

The sphenopalatine foramen, which transmits much of the neurovascular supply to the nasal cavity, is at the posterosuperior corner. The medial pterygoid plates give origin to the fascia and muscle of the wall of the nasopharynx, providing continuity between the nasal cavity and the nasopharynx.

The roof is formed from anterior to posterior by the nasal, frontal (9), cribriform plate of ethmoid (10) and sphenoid (11) bones. The floor is formed by the maxilla (12) and horizontal plate of palatine (13). This horizontal, hard palate separates nasal and oral cavities. Nasogastric tubes must be passed horizontally backward, parallel to the floor of the cavity.

Nasal air sinuses

The frontal, maxilla, ethmoid and sphenoid bones are hollow. The nasal mucous membrane extends into these cavities to form the air-filled nasal sinuses. Their function is uncertain, but they may lighten the skull, add resonance to the voice, and insulate the brain.

Mucus secreted in the sinuses must be carried back into the nasal cavity by the cilia. Should this action be overwhelmed by a common cold, or the sinus openings be obstructed, the mucus may build up and become infected to cause painful sinusitis.

The opening (14) of the maxillary sinus (15) is high up in its medial wall, therefore it is the most difficult to drain, and the one most susceptible to sinusitis. The maxilla houses the upper teeth and their roots may extend into the sinus, creating fistulae following extraction.

The ethmoid is excavated by air cells or sinuses (16) that lie between the lateral wall of the nasal cavity and the medial wall of the orbit. During endoscopic surgery on these sinuses care is taken to avoid arteries passing from the orbit through the ethmoid sinuses into the nasal cavity. The orbit and its contents (particularly the optic nerve) are closely related to the nasal cavity. The pituitary gland (17) lies in its fossa in the sphenoid bone, just above the sphenoidal sinus (18).

Conchae (turbinates) and meati

The three conchae provide a large surface area, slow the air flow, and make it turbulent. The superior (19) and middle (20) conchae are derived from the ethmoid. The inferior concha (21) is a separate bone, fused to the maxilla.

The meati are grooves that lie inferior to each concha. The spheno-ethmoidal recess (22) lies above the variable superior concha to receive the sphenoidal sinus. The superior meatus (23) receives the posterior ethmoidal sinus and the inferior meatus (24) receives the nasolacrimal duct (25).

The middle meatus (26), under the middle concha, shows a bulge caused by the underlying ethmoid (bulla ethmoidalis) (27) and a semicircular groove under the bulge – hiatus semilunaris (29). The frontal sinus opens through the infundibulum anteriorly in the hiatus, whereas the maxillary sinus opens posteriorly. The anterior and middle ethmoid sinuses also open into the middle meatus.

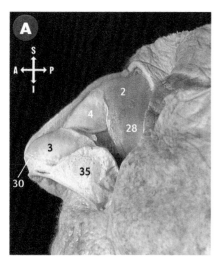

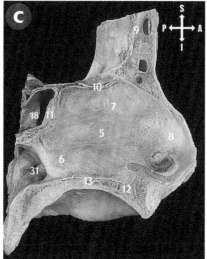

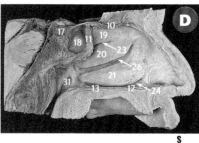

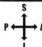

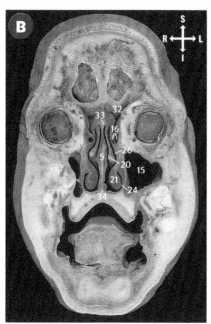

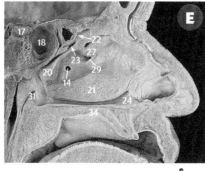

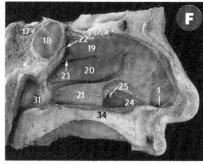

A Cartilages of the external nose (from the left)
B Coronal section through the head (from the front)
C Nasal septum (from the right)
D Lateral wall of the nasal cavity and nasopharynx (from the right)

E Lateral wall of the nasal cavity and semilunar hiatus (from the right)
F Lateral wall of the nasal cavity (from the right)

1	Coarse hairs, vibrissae, in nostril	10	Cribriform plate of ethmoid bone
2	Nasal bone	11	Sphenoid bone
3	Greater nasal cartilage	12	Horizontal plate of maxilla
4	Lateral nasal cartilage	13	Horizontal plate of palatine bone
5	Nasal septum	14	Aperture of maxillary sinus
6	Position of vomer	15	Maxillary sinus
7	Position of perpendicular plate of ethmoid bone	16	Ethmoidal air cells
8	Position of septal cartilage	17	Pituitary gland
9	Frontal bone	18	Sphenoidal sinus
		19	Superior nasal concha
20	Middle nasal concha	29	Semilunar hiatus
21	Inferior nasal concha	30	Septal process (medial crus) of greater nasal cartilage
22	Spheno-ethmoidal recess	31	Opening of auditory (Eustachian) tube
23	Superior meatus	32	Frontal sinus
24	Inferior meatus	33	Roof of nasal cavity
25	Marker within opening of nasolacrimal duct	34	Hard palate
26	Middle meatus	35	Fibrofatty tissue
27	Ethmoidal bulla		
28	Frontal process of maxilla		

Location of numbers: 1F; 2A; 3A; 4A; 5BC; 6C; 7C; 8C; 9C; 10CD; 11CD; 12CD; 13CD; 14E; 15B; 16B; 17DEF; 18CDEF; 19DF; 20BDEF; 21BDEF; 22EF; 23DEF; 24BDEF; 25F; 26BD; 27E; 28A; 29E; 30A; 31CDEF; 32B; 33B; 34BEF; 35A.

Nasopharynx, auditory tube, neurovascular supply of nasal cavity and nasopharynx, maxillary nerve

Nasopharynx – The nasal cavity continues posteriorly into the nasopharynx (1), which is also lined by respiratory epithelium and is held open by the pharyngobasilar fascia that arises from the bones of the skull base. The left and right sides of the pharyngobasilar fascia fuse in the posterior midline and attach to the pharyngeal tubercle about 1 cm anterior to the foramen magnum.

Auditory tube – Equalization of pressure in the middle ear occurs via the auditory (Eustachian) tube (2) that connects the middle ear to the nasopharynx. The tube has a bony part that passes through the petrous temporal bone and a cartilaginous part that lies between the greater wing of sphenoid and the petrous temporal bone. It enters the nasopharynx above the pharyngobasilar fascia. The cartilage forms a tubal eminence (3) and gives partial origin to muscles that elevate the pharynx and soft palate (salpingopharyngeus (4), levator palati (5) and tensor palati (6)). When these muscles contract on swallowing, they open the auditory tube, facilitating the flow of air to and from the middle ear with consequent pressure equalization.

Tonsils – Clusters of lymphoid tissue are gathered under the mucous membrane on the posterior wall of the nasopharynx and around the opening of the auditory tube. These are the pharyngeal (adenoid) (7) and tubal (3) tonsils, which may enlarge following chronic inflammation to obstruct the nasopharynx and auditory tube. The latter may result in recurrent and chronic middle ear infections.

Neurovascular supply of nasal cavity and nasopharynx – Sense of smell is via the olfactory nerves (8,9) that arise in the mucous membrane covering the roof and superior aspects of the lateral walls of the nasal cavity and nasal septum. The nerves pass through the cribriform plate (10) to the olfactory bulbs (11).

Branches of both the ophthalmic (from internal carotid) and maxillary (from external carotid) arteries enter the nasal cavity, accompanying the nerves. There are rich vascular anastomoses, and nosebleeds (epistaxis) are common. Anteriorly, on the septum, the branches from the anterior ethmoidal artery (ophthalmic) anastomose with branches of the sphenopalatine (maxillary). The anastomosis is augmented by incoming branches from the facial artery, and usually also by branches ascending from the palate. This highly vascular spot is Little's area (12) and the most common site of epistaxis, which is treated by packing the nasal cavity. Occasionally the sphenopalatine artery (13), situated posteriorly in the cavity may rupture and bleed profusely. Such haemorrhage may be difficult to control by packing alone and cauterization of vessels or even selective arterial embolization may have to undertaken.

The equivalent nerves are sphenopalatine and nasal branches of the maxillary nerve posteriorly, and anterior ethmoidal branches of the nasociliary (a branch of V^1) anteriorly.

Maxillary nerve (V^2) – The maxillary nerve is a sensory nerve that has 'picked-up' postganglionic secretomotor fibres from the pterygopalatine ganglion. Before passing into the inferior orbital fissure to become the infra-orbital nerve, the maxillary gives a zygomatic branch and the posterior, superior dental (alveolar) nerves. The latter, along with other superior dental nerves that arise from the infra-orbital and pass in the wall of the maxillary sinus (giving the sinus its sensation and secretomotor supply) provide sensation to the upper teeth.

The infra-orbital nerve itself emerges through the infra-orbital foramen to provide sensation to the skin of the lower eyelid and upper lip, and underlying conjunctiva or mucous membrane. The zygomatic branch divides within the orbit into two branches (zygomaticofacial, zygomaticotemporal) that pierce the bone and emerge to give sensation to the skin over the cheekbone and temple, just around the eye. The zygomaticotemporal branch carries the parasympathetic fibres that pass to the lacrimal nerve and give secretomotor supply to the lacrimal gland. The sphenopalatine and nasal branches carry sensation and secretomotor supply to the nasal cavity, both the lateral wall and septum posteriorly. The pharyngeal branch carries the same modalities to the nasopharynx.

The lesser and greater (22) palatine nerves are joined by a few taste fibres. They pass down the palatine canal, and through the greater and lesser palatine foramina to supply the hard and soft palates.

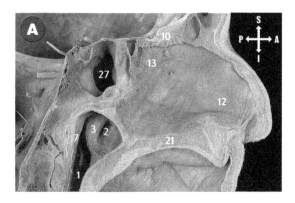

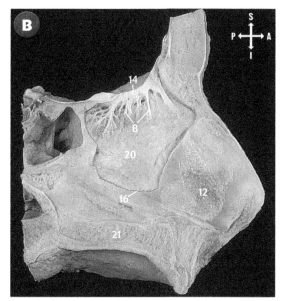

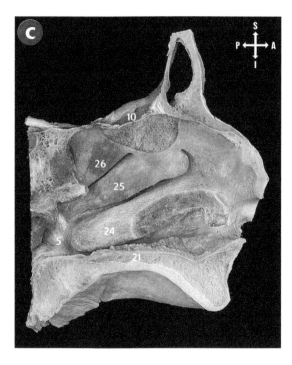

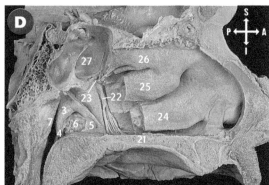

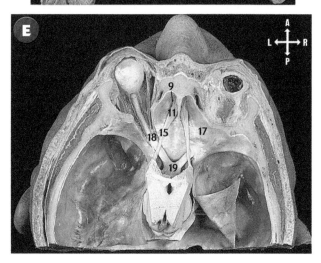

A Nasal septum (from the right)
B Mucous membrane lining of the lateral wall of the nasal septum (from the right)
C Lateral wall of the nasal cavity (from the right)
D Lateral wall of the nasal cavity, palatine canal (from the right)
E Cranial fossae with partial dissection of the left orbit (from above)

1	Nasopharynx (nasal part of pharynx)	7	Position of pharyngeal tonsil (adenoid)
2	Opening of auditory (Eustachian) tube	8	Filaments of olfactory nerve (I)
3	Tubal elevation and position of tubal tonsil	9	Olfactory nerve (I) filaments passing through the cribriform plate of the ethmoid bone within dural sheaths
4	Salpingopharyngeus	10	Cribriform plate of ethmoid bone
5	Levator veli palatini (levator palati)	11	Olfactory bulb
6	Tensor veli palatini (tensor palati)		

12	Position of Little's area
13	Position of sphenopalatine artery
14	Position of olfactory bulb
15	Olfactory tract
16	Cut edge of nasal septum mucosa
17	Dura mater
18	Optic nerve (II)
19	Optic chiasma

20	Perpendicular plate of ethmoid
21	Hard palate
22	Greater palatine nerve and canal
23	Pterygopalatine ganglion
24	Inferior nasal concha
25	Middle nasal concha
26	Superior nasal concha
27	Sphenoidal sinus

Location of numbers: 1A; 2A; 3AD; 4D; 5CD; 6D; 7AD; 8B; 9E; 10AC; 11E; 12AB; 13A; 14B; 15E; 16B; 17E; 18E; 19E; 20B; 21ABCD; 22D; 23D; 24CD; 25CD; 26CD; 27AD.

Temporomandibular joint and muscles

The bony surfaces of the temporomandibular joint (TMJ) are lined by fibrocartilage instead of hyaline cartilage. The head of the mandible (1) articulates with the mandibular fossa. The TMJ is divided into an upper and a lower joint by a fibrocartilaginous disc (2) that sits over the mandibular head, but also attaches to the joint capsule peripherally and into the squamotympanic fissure posteriorly. **The disc may deteriorate, causing pain in the joint.** The capsule attaches to the articular margins (anterior to the articular tubercle) and thickens laterally as the strong, lateral temporomandibular ligament (3). There are two associated ligaments that are separate from the joint: sphenomandibular, from spine of sphenoid to lingula of mandible; stylomandibular (4), from styloid process to angle of mandible.

Movements of the temporomandibular joint

The inferior alveolar (dental) nerve enters the mandible through the mandibular foramen, posteromedial to the lingula. To prevent stretching of the nerve during opening of the mouth, the axis of this movement passes through the lingulae. When opening the mouth, the head of the mandible and its overlying disc are drawn forward and downward onto the articular tubercle (protrusion). There is associated rotation of the mandibular head in relation to the disc for further mandibular depression and wider opening of the mouth. Protrusion takes place in the upper joint cavity, which is lax enough to allow this. As a result, **it is possible to dislocate the TMJ anteriorly if the mouth is opened too widely.** To close the mouth, the head of the mandible and disc must be retracted back into the mandibular fossa, and the mandible elevated by rotation.

When chewing food, the mandible tends to swing from side to side by the following repeated mechanism. The left mandibular head is held in the fossa. The right head is protruded, then retracted and held, while the left head is protruded and then retracted. During protrusion, as the head and disc slide down the articular tubercle, the teeth separate. During chewing this must be counteracted by rotatory mandibular elevation.

Muscles of mastication (all supplied by V³)

Opening the mouth. Lateral pterygoid (5) arises from the lateral aspect of the lateral pterygoid plate and the roof of the infratemporal fossa. The fibres pass posteriorly to insert into the mandibular condyle, the capsule and the disc of the TMJ. The muscle draws the condyle and disc forward and down the articular tubercle in protrusion. Lateral pterygoid is the only primary muscle of mastication that opens the mouth. Muscles passing upward from the hyoid to the mandible, in particular digastric (6), may assist it.

Closing the mouth. The three other primary muscles of mastication elevate the mandible in biting, chewing and grinding. Their resting tone maintains normal closure of the mouth. Temporalis (7,8) arises from the temporal fossa and overlying fascia. It passes deep to the zygomatic arch to attach to the coronoid process (9) and anterior aspect of the mandibular ramus. Its posterior, horizontal fibres retract the mandible. The anterior ones are powerful elevators.

Masseter (10) passes from the zygomatic arch (11) to the lateral aspect of the mandibular ramus. Medial pterygoid (12) is a deeper, almost mirror image of masseter. It arises from the lateral pterygoid plate, but from its medial aspect. There is a small superficial head from the maxilla. It inserts onto the medial aspect of the mandibular ramus. Both masseter and medial pterygoid are powerful elevators of the mandible and both aid protrusion as their fibres pass slightly posteriorly as well as inferiorly.

The maxillary artery (13), a terminal branch of the external carotid, arises in the parotid gland to pass anteriorly deep to the neck of the mandible (15). In the infratemporal fossa it sends branches to the masticatory muscles, to the external acoustic meatus and to the middle ear. The middle meningeal artery also arises here and pierces the auriculotemporal nerve before entering the skull. The maxillary artery then sends branches to pass with all the branches of the mandibular nerve, e.g. lingual (16) and inferior alveolar (17), before passing through the pterygomaxillary fissure to enter the pterygopalatine fossa. It then sends branches with all those of the maxillary nerve and pterygopalatine ganglion.

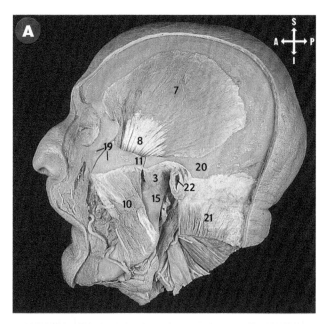

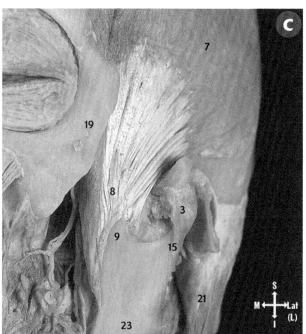

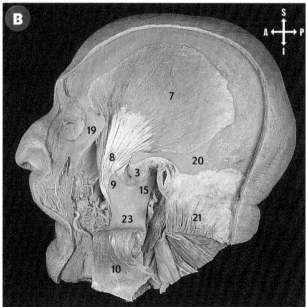

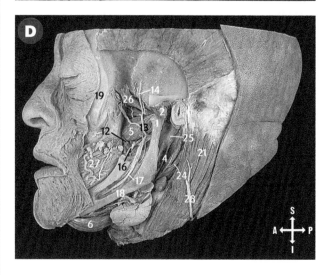

A Side of face, muscles of mastication (from the left)
B Side of face, temporomandibular joint (from the left)

C Side of face, temporalis tendon (from the front and left)
D Side of face, infratemporal fossa (from the left)

1 Head of mandible	**7** Temporalis	**15** Neck of mandible	**23** Ramus of mandible
2 Articular disc of temporomandibular joint	**8** Temporalis tendon	**16** Lingual nerve	**24** Posterior belly of digastric
3 Lateral ligament of temporomandibular joint	**9** Coronoid process of mandible	**17** Inferior alveolar nerve	**25** Styloid process
4 Stylomandibular ligament	**10** Masseter	**18** Body of mandible	**26** Upper head of lateral pterygoid
5 Lower head of lateral pterygoid	**11** Zygomatic arch	**19** Zygomatic bone	**27** Buccinator
6 Anterior belly of digastric	**12** Medial pterygoid	**20** Temporal bone	**28** Great auricular nerve
	13 Maxillary artery	**21** Sternocleidomastoid	
	14 Deep temporal artery	**22** External acoustic meatus	

Location of numbers: 1D; **2**D; **3**ABC; **4**D; **5**D; **6**D; **7**ABC; **8**ABC; **9**BC; **10**AB; **11**A; **12**D; **13**D; **14**D; **15**ABC; **16**D; **17**D; **18**D; **19**ABCD; **20**AB; **21**ABCD; **22**A; **23**BC; **24**D; **25**D; **26**D; **27**D; **28**D.

Face: skeleton, muscles; scalp

The face is dominated by the orbital, nasal and oral cavities, each having groups of sphincter and dilator muscles. The muscles around the oral cavity are important when eating, and all the muscles insert into the overlying skin as muscles of facial expression. The scalp is essential for some facial expressions. Words and speech are formed by movement of the lips and cheeks as well as the tongue. Any injury affecting the facial muscles or their nerve supply (VII) may well affect facial movements and speech. Therefore the motor and sensory nerve supplies to this region are important in clinical examination.

Five layers of the scalp

1 – The skin (1) has hair and associated sebaceous glands, which may form cysts. Cutaneous nerves derived from the V^1, V^3 and the occipital nerves converge into the scalp from the periphery.

2 – The subcutaneous tissue connects the skin to the underlying aponeurosis. It is dense, thick tissue with a rich blood supply. The arteries anastomose freely from both sides and from branches of both the internal and external carotids. The rich anastomosis and dense connective tissue that tends to hold open a lacerated artery means scalp wounds bleed profusely. When carrying out neurosurgery the scalp must be lifted, usually on the vascular pedicle of the superficial temporal artery (10). Venous drainage from the forehead passes via ophthalmic veins into the cavernous sinuses and forms a possible route for spread of infection to those sinuses.

3 – Occipitalis (2) has a muscle belly on each side that arises from the skull and inserts into the epicranial aponeurosis (3). The aponeurosis gives origin to frontalis (4), which anteriorly attaches to the skin of the eyebrow. Laterally the aponeurosis thins and blends with the fascia over temporalis (6). Together occipitalis and frontalis contract to raise the eyebrows. Frontalis contracts to frown or wrinkle the forehead.

4 – The loose connective tissue beneath the aponeurosis allows the scalp movement described above. It may also allow traumatic lifting of the scalp, e.g. should long hair be caught in machinery. Following wounds to the scalp foreign bodies may enter this layer.

5 – The periosteum (7) adheres to the bone and is continuous with the periosteal layer of dura mater at the foramina and via the sutures.

Muscles around the oral cavity

Buccinator (12) compresses the cheeks to keep food between the teeth when chewing. It arises from the maxilla and mandible, away from the alveolar bone that supports the teeth. As the fibres pass backward they pass medially behind the upper and lower molar teeth to merge with the superior constrictor muscle of the pharynx and form the pterygomandibular raphe that ensures continuity of the cheeks and pharynx.

As the fibres of buccinator pass forward into the lips they form orbicularis oris (13). The central fibres cross each other so that lower central fibres go to the upper lip and upper central fibres to the lower lip, forming the modiolus (14) just lateral to the corner of the mouth. The upper and lower fibres of buccinator pass into the upper and lower lips, respectively. As a result, orbicularis oris encircles the lips and is the sphincter that keeps them closed when chewing.

The dilator muscles (15,16) meet at the modiolus and usually contribute to orbicularis oris. These four muscles have the actions implied by their names: levator and depressor anguli; levator and depressor labii. Two (often variable) zygomatic muscles (17) arise from the zygoma and pass to the upper lip and angle of the mouth. Along with risorius, which arises from the parotid fascia and goes to the skin of the angle of the mouth, they contribute to smiling and grinning. Mentalis (18) pulls the skin upward to help protrude the lower lip in drinking and pouting.

Platysma (19) lies in the superficial fascia and is highly variable. It passes from the upper thoracic wall, through the neck and into the lower lip, with a few fibres attaching to the mandible. It depresses the lower lip in a grimace and also prevents indrawing if the structures in the neck during forced inspiratory effort.

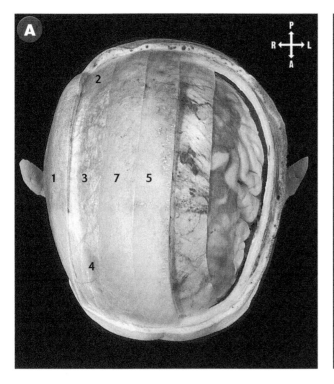

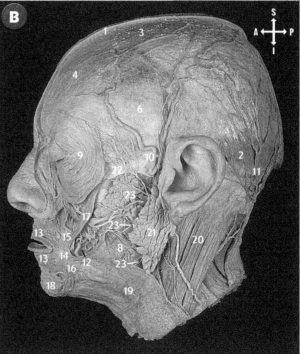

A Cranial vault, stepped dissection (from above)
B Side of face, superficial dissection (from the left)

1	Skin and dense subcutaneous tissue		occipitofrontalis)	
2	Occipitalis (occipital belly of occipitofrontalis)	5	Bone of cranial vault	
3	Epicranial aponeurosis (galea aponeurotica)	6	Temporal fascia	
4	Frontalis (frontal belly of	7	Loose connective tissue and pericranium (periosteum)	

1 Skin and dense subcutaneous tissue
2 Occipitalis (occipital belly of occipitofrontalis)
3 Epicranial aponeurosis (galea aponeurotica)
4 Frontalis (frontal belly of occipitofrontalis)
5 Bone of cranial vault
6 Temporal fascia
7 Loose connective tissue and pericranium (periosteum)
8 Masseter
9 Orbicularis oculi
10 Superficial temporal artery
11 Occipital artery
12 Buccinator
13 Orbicularis oris
14 Modiolus
15 Levator anguli oris
16 Depressor anguli oris
17 Zygomaticus major
18 Mentalis
19 Platysma
20 Sternocleidomastoid
21 Parotid gland
22 Zygomatic arch
23 Facial nerve branches

Location of numbers: **1**AB; **2**AB; **3**AB; **4**AB; **5**A; **6**B; **7**A; **8**B; **9**B; **10**B; **11**B; **12**B; **13**B; **14**B; **15**B; **16**B; **17**B; **18**B; **19**B; **20**B; **21**B; **22**B; **23**B.

Facial neurovascular supply, salivary glands

The facial nerve passes through the middle ear to emerge from the stylomastoid foramen. It supplies occipitalis (1), posterior belly of digastric and stylohyoid before entering the parotid gland (2). It branches variably within the gland, but the more frequent appearance is of five branches splaying across the face: temporal (3) to frontalis; zygomatic (4) to orbicularis oculi; buccal (5) to buccinator and muscles of the upper lip; marginal mandibular (6) to muscles of the lower lip; and cervical (7) to platysma.

The marginal mandibular branch dips below the mandible to overly the submandibular gland (8), where it is susceptible during gland surgery. Injury causes lower lip paralysis and saliva dribbles from the mouth. The mastoid process (9) is not formed at birth and the facial nerve may be injured during forceps delivery. Similarly, the nerve may be injured just before emerging from the stylomastoid foramen. Such diseases (Bell's palsy) show weakness of all the muscles from frontalis to platysma, on the ipsilateral side of the face. A cerebrovascular accident affecting one half of the brain will not affect the upper face, but will weaken the lower opposite facial muscles. Consequently, all aspects of facial muscle function must be clinically assessed.

Sensory nerve supply of the facial skin

The skin over the angle of the mandible (10) is supplied by C2,3 via the great auricular nerve (11). The remainder is via branches of the trigeminal nerve:

- Upper eyelid, forehead to vertex, root and tip of nose – ophthalmic via lacrimal, supra-orbital, supra-trochlear and nasociliary.
- Lower eye lid, upper lip, upper cheek – maxillary via infra-orbital, zygomaticotemporal and zygomaticofacial.
- Lower lip, chin, lower cheek, temporal region – mandibular via mental, buccal, and auriculotemporal.

Each region of nerve distribution may be individually affected by shingles or by trigeminal neuralgia and should be tested individually. Shingles seen on the tip of the nose may also affect the cornea as branches of the nasociliary nerve supply both. Sensory supply to eyelid, lip and cheek is the same for skin and underlying mucous membrane.

Blood supply

The facial artery (12), branch of external carotid, is palpable as it passes over the mandible, anterior to masseter (13). The left and right facial arteries anastomose freely. Veins converge on the facial vein (14), which joins the internal jugular. There may be deep connections to the cavernous sinus via the venous plexus around the pterygoid muscles (route for spread of infection).

Salivary glands

Saliva wets and lubricates food; it also contains enzymes to commence digestion. Small salivary glands are scattered under the mucous membrane of the lips and cheeks, and the sublingual glands (Illustration G) lie under the tongue, on the floor of the mouth. The parotid (Illustration F) secretes serous saliva, and the submandibular (Illustration E) secretes seromucous saliva.

The parotid lies between the mastoid process and the mandibular ramus. It overlaps sternocleidomastoid (15) and masseter, and extends medially as far as the styloid process (16). The facial nerve lies lateral to the retromandibular vein and external carotid artery within the gland, which is enclosed in deep fascia, therefore swelling of the gland and its associated lymph nodes (mumps) is painful. The secretomotor supply is from the glossopharyngeal, via the auriculotemporal nerve. The parotid duct (17) crosses masseter where there may be a small accessory parotid lobe (18) superior to it. The duct pierces buccinator to enter the oral cavity opposite the second upper molar tooth. It takes an oblique course through buccinator, creating a sphincteric affect.

The submandibular gland lies inferior to the body of the mandible, between it and mylohyoid (19). It curves around the posterior aspect of mylohyoid to lie between it and hyoglossus (20). From this deeper part of the gland, the submandibular duct (21) passes forward (surrounded by the sublingual gland (22) and receiving its ducts) to open on the sublingual papilla (40) on the lingual frenulum. The secretomotor supply for both glands is via chorda tympani (VII), running with the lingual nerve that winds inferior to, and then medial to, the submandibular duct before passing upward to the tongue. Stones within the submandibular duct cause obstruction and painful swelling of the gland on salivation.

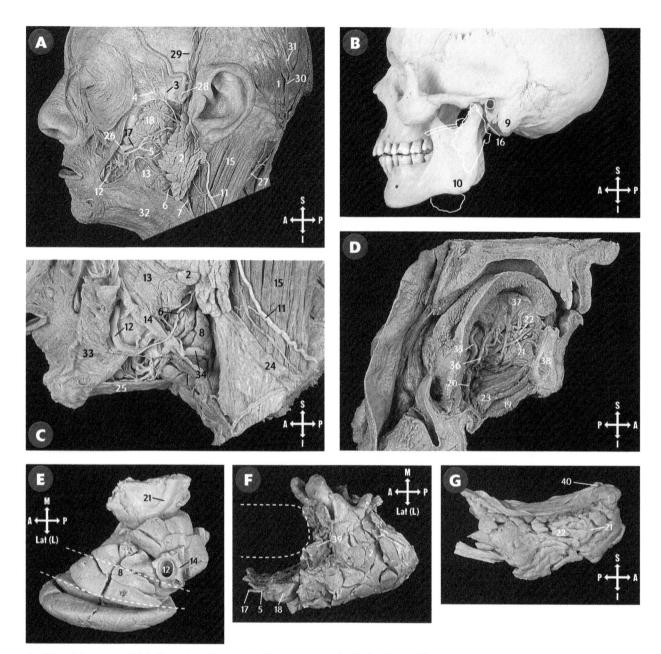

A Side of face superficial dissection (from the left)
B Skull with mandible (from the left) with outline position
of parotid gland and duct, and submandibular gland
C Left side of face, submandibular region (from the left)
D Deep dissection of the tongue (from the right)

E Left submandibular gland with outline position of
mandible (from above)
F Left parotid gland with outline position of mandible
(from above)
G Left sublingual gland (from the right)

1	Occipitalis (occipital belly of occipitofrontalis)	10	Angle of mandible
2	Parotid gland	11	Great auricular nerve
3	Temporal branches of VII	12	Facial artery
4	Zygomatic branches of VII	13	Masseter
5	Buccal branches of VII	14	Facial vein
6	Marginal mandibular branches of VII	15	Sternocleidomastoid
7	Cervical branches of VII	16	Styloid process
8	Submandibular gland	17	Parotid duct
9	Mastoid process	18	Accessory lobe of parotid gland
		19	Mylohyoid
		20	Hyoglossus

21	Submandibular duct
22	Sublingual gland
23	Geniohyoid
24	External jugular vein
25	Anterior belly of digastric
26	Buccal fat pad
27	Lesser occipital nerve
28	Superficial temporal artery
29	Auriculotemporal nerve
30	Occipital artery
31	Greater occipital nerve

32	Platysma
33	Platysma (reflected)
34	Lymph node
35	Lingual artery
36	Lingual nerve
37	Genioglossus anterior part
38	Body of mandible
39	Maxillary artery
40	Orifice of submandibular duct (sublingual papilla)

Location of numbers: **1**A; **2**ACF; **3**A; **4**A; **5**AF; **6**AC; **7**A; **8**CE; **9**B; **10**B; **11**AC; **12**ACE; **13**AC; **14**CE; **15**AC; **16**B; **17**AF; **18**AF; **19**D; **20**D; **21**DEG; **22**DG; **23**D; **24**C; **25**C; **26**A; **27**A; **28**A; **29**A; **30**A; **31**A; **32**A; **33**C; **34**C; **35**D; **36**D; **37**D; **38**D; **39**F; **40**G.

Oral cavity, teeth, tongue

The maxillae (Illustration C, 1) and mandible (Illustration D, 2) support the oral cavity, for drinking, eating, chewing and speech. The oral cavity lies between the cheeks and lips, which are formed by skin and mucous membrane with muscle between. The oral cavity proper is internal to the teeth. The vestibule is outside the teeth and compressed by buccinator and orbicularis oris. Posteriorly, the cavity is continuous with the oropharynx (3). The hard (4) and soft (5) palates form the roof. The floor comprises mylohyoid muscle (6), which arises from the inner aspect of the mandible to fuse with its neighbour in the midline, forming a central raphe from mandible to hyoid (7). Further support and control of the floor of the mouth, and therefore the tongue, is provided by geniohyoid (8), internal to mylohyoid, and by the anterior belly of digastric external to it.

Mylohyoid and hyoglossus (9) lie opposed to each other. The lingual nerve (10), submandibular duct (11) and hypoglossal nerve (12) enter the oral cavity between them. The lingual artery (13) and glossopharyngeal nerve (14) enter deep to hyoglossus.

Infections, usually from tooth abscesses, may track backward in the fascial planes between the muscles, and then around the pharynx or toward the larynx. Such infections require urgent treatment to prevent dangerous spread, or life-threatening laryngeal oedema.

Teeth

The teeth cut, tear and grind food. They are held by the periodontal ligament in the alveolar bone at the margins of both jaws. Two identical sets of eight teeth

in each jaw makes thirty-two altogether. Third molars (wisdom teeth) may erupt at an angle causing impaction, necessitating extraction. Alveolar bone resorbs following tooth loss or extraction.

Superior alveolar (dental) branches of the maxillary and infra-orbital nerves supply the upper teeth and

gums. The maxilla is relatively thin and anaesthetic injected into the gum will anaesthetize the dental nerves. As the superior alveolar nerves also supply the maxillary sinus, sinusitis may mimic toothache. The inferior alveolar (dental) branch of V³ supplies all the lower teeth and then gives off the mental nerve through the mental foramen to supply the skin of the chin, the lower lip and its underlying mucous membrane. The inferior alveolar continues in the bone as the incisive nerve to the incisor teeth, sometimes crossing the midline. Anaesthetic may be injected via the mental foramen to anaesthetize the incisive nerve. The buccal nerve supplies the gums lateral to the molars and must be anaesthetized directly.

Tongue

The tongue is for manipulating food, and for speech. It is formed by muscles enclosed by mucous membrane continuous with the floor of the mouth and covered with stratified squamous epithelium.

Intrinsic muscles run in different directions completely within the tongue and alter its shape. Extrinsic muscles pass into the tongue from surrounding bones, and alter its position during chewing and swallowing. Genioglossus (20) draws the tongue downward and forward. Hyoglossus pulls the sides of the tongue downward. Palatoglossus and styloglossus pass downward and forward into the tongue from the palate and styloid process, respectively. They pull the tongue upward and backward in swallowing.

Palatoglossus raises folds, one on each side, the pillars of the fauces (21). They separate the oral cavity from the oropharynx. While chewing, the pillars approximate to each other, and to the soft palate, to prevent food entering the pharynx, and possibly the larynx during inspiration. The hypoglossal supplies all the tongue muscles except palatoglossus, which is supplied by the pharyngeal plexus.

The mucous membrane under the tongue and on the floor of the mouth is smooth, and its sensory supply is by the lingual nerve. The dorsum of the tongue is divided by the sulcus terminalis (22) into anterior two-thirds and posterior one-third. The former is covered by filiform papillae giving the tongue its 'furry' appearance and helping grasp food. Fungiform papillae (23), with taste buds, are scattered around the tongue surface. The circumvallate papillae (24), also with taste buds, lie in front of the sulcus terminalis. The lingual nerve, which has the chorda tympani running with it to supply taste sensation, supplies general sensation to the anterior two-thirds. The posterior one-third is supplied by glossopharyngeal for both general sensation and taste.

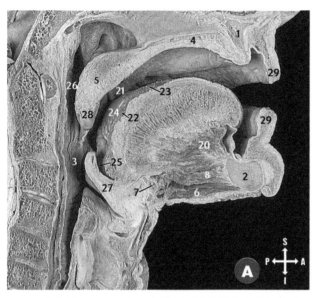

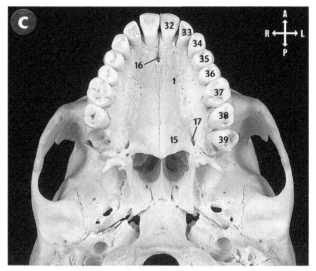

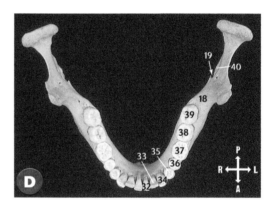

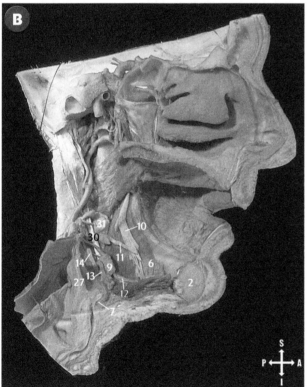

A Midline sagittal section through the mouth (from the right)
B Deep dissection of the floor of the mouth (from the right)
C Skull, dentition (from below)
D Mandible, dentition (from above)

1	Maxilla	**11**	Submandibular duct	
2	Body of mandible	**12**	Hypoglossal nerve	
3	Oropharynx (oral part of pharynx)	**13**	Lingual artery	
4	Hard palate	**14**	Glossopharyngeal nerve	
5	Soft palate	**15**	Horizontal plate of palatine bone	
6	Mylohyoid	**16**	Incisive foramen	
7	Body of hyoid bone	**17**	Greater palatine foramen	
8	Geniohyoid	**18**	Retromolar fossa of mandible	
9	Hyoglossus	**19**	Mandibular foramen	
10	Lingual nerve	**20**	Genioglossus	

21	Palatoglossal fold (pillars of fauces)	**31**	Deep part of submandibular gland
22	Sulcus terminalis	**32**	Central incisor
23	Fungiform papillae	**33**	Lateral incisor
24	Vallate papillae	**34**	Canine
25	Vallecula	**35**	First premolar
26	Nasopharynx (nasal part of pharynx)	**36**	Second premolar
27	Epiglottis	**37**	First molar
28	Uvula	**38**	Second molar
29	Lip	**39**	Third molar
30	Tendon of digastric	**40**	Angle of mandible

Location of numbers: **1**AC; **2**AB; **3**A; **4**A; **5**A; **6**AB; **7**AB; **8**A; **9**B; **10**B; **11**B; **12**B; **13**B; **14**B; **15**C; **16**C; **17**C; **18**D; **19**D; **20**A; **21**A; **22**A; **23**A; **24**A; **25**A; **26**A; **27**AB; **28**A; **29**A; **30**B; **31**B; **32**CD; **33**CD; **34**CD; **35**CD; **36**CD; **37**CD; **38**CD; **39**CD; **40**D.

Soft palate, tonsils, pharynx

The palate is overlain by mucous membrane with stratified squamous epithelium. The sensory and secretomotor supply is mainly via the greater and lesser palatine nerves, with the sphenopalatine anteriorly.

The soft palate (1) is tensed during swallowing and elevated to lie in a 'socket' (created by a few circular fibres of palatopharyngeus) and separate the oropharynx (2) from the nasopharynx (3). It is formed by the aponeuroses of the tensor palati muscles. Each of these arises from a fossa in the sphenoid, immediately medial to the foramen ovale (the emerging mandibular nerve lies on the lateral surface of tensor palati). The muscle belly then lies between the lateral and medial pterygoid plates. Its tendon hooks around the pterygoid hamulus at the inferior end of the medial pterygoid plate, and flares into a flat, triangular aponeurosis that attaches to the palatine bone anteriorly and its neighbour from the opposite side medially. The aponeurosis is covered by a glandular mucous membrane that forms the dependent uvula (4). Tensor palati is supplied by V³. Levator palati (5) arises within the pharynx from the apex of the petrous temporal bone and passes inferiorly to insert into the palatine aponeurosis.

Tonsils

The lingual tonsil (6) lies under the mucous membrane of the posterior one-third of the tongue. The palatine tonsil (7) lies in the fossa behind palatoglossus, but in front of palatopharyngeus (8).

Tonsils are clusters of lymphocytes, but the overlying mucous membrane dips into the tonsillar tissue to form crypts. The lingual, palatine, pharyngeal and tubal tonsils form a protective lymphoid ring around the entries to the respiratory and digestive tracts. The bed of the palatine tonsil is highly vascular, receiving branches from the facial artery. Occasionally, there can be considerable bleeding during or following excision of the tonsil. The mucous membrane overlying the palatine tonsil is supplied by a plexus that includes the maxillary and glossopharyngeal nerves. The glossopharyngeal also supplies the middle ear therefore tonsillitis may refer pain to the middle ear.

Pharynx

The pharynx is for the passage of air from the nasal cavity to the larynx and trachea, and for food from the oral cavity to the laryngopharynx (9) and oesophagus. The oropharynx is a passage for food or air, depending on the position of the soft palate. The pharyngobasilar fascia (10) holds the nasopharynx open, but the constrictor muscles help squeeze a bolus of food inferiorly toward the oesophagus.

Superior constrictor (11) arises from the medial pterygoid plate and the pterygomandibular raphe, which ensures continuity between it and buccinator. Middle constrictor (12) arises from the hyoid bone and stylohyoid ligament. Inferior constrictor arises from the thyroid and cricoid cartilages: thyropharyngeus (13) and cricopharyngeus (14). The constrictors sweep around the pharynx and fuse in the pharyngeal raphe (15). They overlap each other and the pharyngobasilar fascia so that much of the pharynx has three layers in its wall. More inferiorly, there may be only middle and inferior constrictors, leaving a possible weakness in the wall and the potential for the formation of a pharyngeal diverticulum (pouch). Cricopharyngeus forms a sphincteric ring around the lower pharynx and is only open during swallowing. Otherwise air would be sucked into the oesophagus during thoracic expansion for inhalation.

On swallowing, the pharynx is elevated to meet the bolus by muscles arising from the skull and descending to merge with the constrictors and the mucous membrane. The site of origin is implied by their names: salpingopharyngeus (16) from the cartilage of the auditory tube; palatopharyngeus from the palate; stylopharyngeus from the styloid process. Pharyngeal elevation also causes simultaneous elevation of the larynx, which is vital for laryngeal closure, and the prevention of food or fluid entering the airway during swallowing.

The pharyngeal plexus gives sensory supply to the oropharynx and motor supply to all the above muscles except tensor palati (V³) and stylopharyngeus (IX). The plexus is composed of: sensory fibres from the glossopharyngeal; sympathetic fibres from the sympathetic trunk; somatic motor and parasympathetic secretomotor fibres from the vagus. Sensation to the mucous membrane of the pharynx is supplied by: the pharyngeal branch of the maxillary, to nasopharynx; the glossopharyngeal via the pharyngeal plexus, to oropharynx; the vagus, to laryngopharynx.

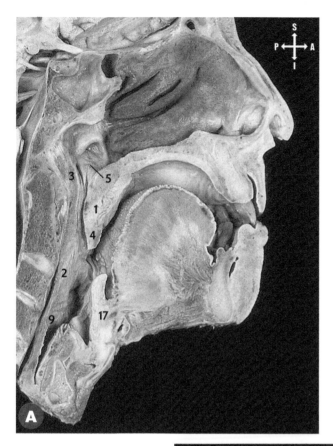

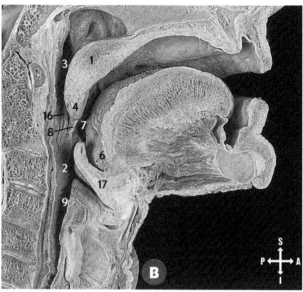

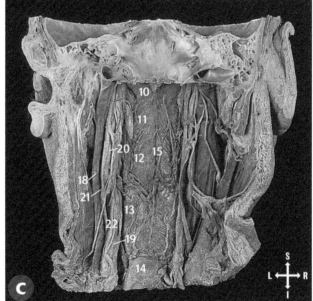

A Mouth and pharynx (from the right)

B Mouth and pharynx (from the right)

C Pharynx (from behind)

1	Soft palate	**6**	Lingual tonsil	**12**	Middle constrictor	**16** Position of salpingopharyngeus
2	Oropharynx (oral part of pharynx)	**7**	Palatine tonsil	**13**	Thyropharyngeus part of inferior constrictor	**17** Epiglottis
3	Nasopharynx (nasal part of pharynx)	**8**	Palatopharyngeus			**18** Internal jugular vein
4	Uvula	**9**	Laryngopharynx (laryngeal part of pharynx)	**14**	Cricopharyngeus part of inferior constrictor	**19** Common carotid artery
5	Position of levator veli palati (tensor veli palatini)	**10**	Pharyngobasilar fascia	**15**	Posterior, midline, pharyngeal raphe	**20** Internal carotid artery
		11	Superior constrictor			**21** Vagus nerve (X)
						22 Sympathetic chain

Location of numbers: 1AB; **2**AB; **3**AB; **4**AB; **5**A; **6**B; **7**B; **8**B; **9**AB; **10**C; **11**C; **12**C; **13**C; **14**C; **15**C; **16**B; **17**AB; **18**C; **19**C; **20**C; **21**C; **22**C.

Larynx, trachea

The inlet of the larynx is a sphincter to protect the airway. The vocal cords act in phonation, coughing, sneezing and raising intra-abdominal pressure. Like all conductive parts of the airway, the larynx must be held open. Other functions depend on alteration of the airway diameter, so the larynx is composed of fibro-elastic membranes suspended between cartilages joined to each other and controlled by muscles. The passages are lined by respiratory epithelium.

The laryngeal inlet opens posteriorly and slightly superiorly into the pharynx. The piriform fossae (1) lie between the sidewalls of the larynx and of the pharynx. The valleculae lie between the tongue and the epiglottis (2). Foreign bodies may be caught in the valleculae and/or piriform fossae.

The hyoid bone (3) is attached to the superior horn (4) of the thyroid cartilage. The laryngeal cartilages are all hyaline, except the epiglottis, which is elastic. The thyroid cartilage (5) has a notch (6) superiorly. It is palpable in the neck, as is the hyoid, and both may be felt moving upward on swallowing. The epiglottis attaches to the thyroid cartilage and extends upward, anteriorly in the larynx and pharynx, but posterior to the tongue. During swallowing it is pushed backward like a lid over the closed laryngeal inlet. The epiglottis is not essential for laryngeal closure.

The cricoid cartilage has a lamina (7) and an arch (8). It is the only complete ring in the airway. The arytenoid cartilages (9) are pyramidal, and sit on the 'shoulders' of the cricoid lamina. Both have an anterior, vocal process that extends into the vocal fold (10) and a lateral, muscular process (11), for insertion of some of the muscles that move them.

Laryngeal membranes

The thyrohyoid membrane lies between the hyoid bone and the thyroid cartilage. The internal laryngeal branches of the superior laryngeal neurovascular bundle pierce it. The quadrangular membrane has an upper edge, the aryepiglottic fold, running upward obliquely from the arytenoid to the epiglottis. This fold, with its neighbour on the other side, forms the laryngeal inlet. The lower edge of the quadrangular membrane runs from the arytenoid to the thyroid cartilage to form the vestibular or false vocal fold (12).

The cricothyroid membrane is suspended between the cricoid and thyroid cartilages, but extends upward to the vocal process of the arytenoid. Its upper free edge passes from the vocal process to the thyroid cartilage as the true vocal fold. The lower edge fuses with the cricoid ring. Anteriorly the cricothyroid membranes fuse and are palpable between the thyroid and cricoid cartilages. Laryngeal inflammation and consequent oedema may completely obstruct the airway. This is life-threatening and must be rapidly recognized so that an opening may be made urgently below the obstruction (cricothyroidotomy (13)).

The ventricle or sinus of the larynx lies between the vestibular and vocal folds. Here the mucous membrane bulges upward as a saccule outside the quadrangular membrane. The saccule is lined by mucus-secreting epithelium to lubricate the vocal folds.

Trachea

The trachea continues from the larynx at C6, through the neck into the thorax where it divides to form the right and left main bronchi to carry air to and from the lungs. It is a fibro-elastic and muscular tube, held open by sixteen to twenty C-shaped rings of hyaline cartilage (14) and lined by respiratory epithelium. Cigarette smoking paralyses the cilia, debilitating the normal mechanism of mucus removal from the respiratory system.

The C-shaped cartilages are deficient posteriorly where the trachea is related to the oesophagus – their ends joined by trachealis (15) muscle to control tracheal diameter. It is narrowed in coughing and to decrease respiratory dead space, but opens to facilitate improved airflow. The elasticity of the trachea allows stretching during swallowing or inhalation, followed by elastic recoil.

Tracheostomy (16) is carried out electively by removing parts of the second and third tracheal cartilages. Care must be taken to avoid the inferior thyroid veins that pass inferiorly in the midline.

Tracheal blood supply is via inferior thyroid and bronchial vessels. Lymph drains to tracheobronchial and paratracheal nodes. Sensory and secretomotor supply is via the recurrent laryngeal nerves.

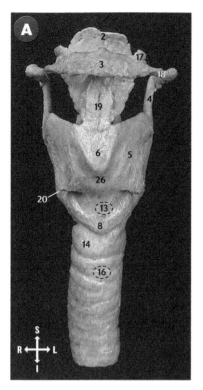

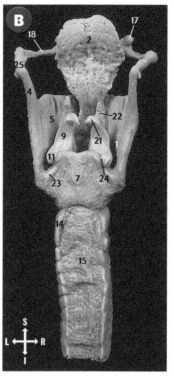

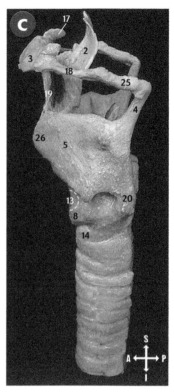

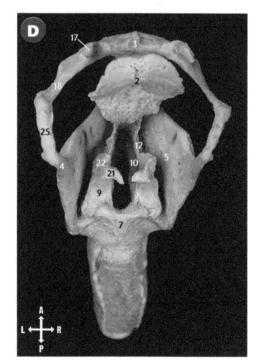

A Hyoid bone and cartilages of the larynx (from the front)
B Hyoid bone and cartilages of the larynx (from behind)
C Hyoid bone and cartilages of the larynx (from the left)
D Hyoid bone and cartilages of the larynx (from above and behind)

1 Piriform fossa (recess)	**7** Lamina of cricoid cartilage	**13** Site of cricothyroidotomy	**20** Inferior horn of thyroid cartilage
2 Epiglottis	**8** Arch of cricoid cartilage	**14** First tracheal ring	**21** Corniculate cartilage
3 Body of hyoid bone	**9** Arytenoid cartilage	**15** Trachealis	**22** Cuneiform cartilage
4 Superior horn of thyroid cartilage	**10** Vocal ligament (true vocal cord)	**16** Site of tracheostomy	**23** Cricothyroid joint
	11 Muscular process of arytenoid cartilage	**17** Lesser horn of hyoid bone	**24** Crico-arytenoid joint
5 Lamina of thyroid cartilage	**12** Vestibular fold (false vocal cord)	**18** Greater horn of hyoid bone	**25** Lateral thyrohyoid ligament
6 Thyroid notch		**19** Median thyrohyoid membrane	**26** Laryngeal prominence

Location of numbers: 1B; 2ABCD; 3ACD; 4ABCD; 5ABCD; 6A; 7BD; 8AC; 9BD; 10D; 11B; 12D; 13AC; 14ABC; 15B; 16A; 17ABCD; 18ABCD; 19A; 20AC; 21BD; 22BD; 23B; 24B; 25BCD; 26AC.

Laryngeal muscles

The extrinsic laryngeal muscles attach the larynx to neighbouring structures and are important laryngeal elevators. The hyoid bone attaches to the larynx, and the pharyngeal inferior constrictor (8) arises from the laryngeal cartilages, so any muscles that elevate the hyoid and pharynx will elevate the larynx.

During swallowing the laryngeal inlet must close. The tongue is pulled upward and backward to tip the bolus into the pharynx. The pharynx and larynx are elevated. Geniohyoid pulls the larynx slightly forward as well as upward, therefore, it is effectively pulled upward under the back of the tongue. This is the main contributor to closure of the laryngeal inlet. The intrinsic muscles alter the diameters within the larynx: open or close the inlet; open or close the vocal folds; lengthen or shorten the vocal folds.

The inlet is closed by laryngeal elevation, aided by the oblique arytenoid (9) continuing as aryepiglotticus (10). This muscle arises from the muscular process of one arytenoid, passes upward and medially to wind around the apex of the other arytenoid, and pass in the aryepiglottic fold to the epiglottis. Contraction of these two muscles draws the arytenoids, epiglottis and aryepiglottic folds together in a 'purse string' mechanism to close the inlet. The inlet opens or widens by elastic recoil in the trachea, and gravity causing the larynx to fall inferiorly after swallowing. Thyro-epiglotticus arises from inside the thyroid cartilage to pass upward and medially into the quadrangular membrane. It pulls the aryepiglottic folds open.

Opening (abduction) of the vocal fold is by posterior crico-arytenoid (11), which arises from the cricoid cartilage and inserts into the muscular process of the arytenoid. It has two actions, to pull the arytenoid laterally down the shoulders of the cricoid, and to rotate the muscular process posteriorly so that the vocal process swivels laterally. The two actions open the rima glottidis, the space between the vocal folds. Closure (adduction) of the vocal fold is by two muscles, to counteract the two actions of posterior crico-arytenoid. Transverse arytenoid (12) pulls the two arytenoids medially. Lateral crico-arytenoid passes from the cricoid arch to the muscular process of the arytenoid. It pulls the process anteriorly, to swivel the vocal process medially.

Lengthening of the vocal fold is by cricothyroid (13), which lies between the cricoid arch and the thyroid lamina. It rocks the thyroid forward to increase the distance between it and the arytenoid, therefore increasing vocal fold length to raise the pitch of the voice. Shortening the vocal fold to decrease the pitch is by thyro-arytenoid, which lies within the vocal fold and draws the thyroid and arytenoid toward each other. Vocalis is a subsidiary muscle within the vocal fold and alters its thickness.

All the laryngeal muscles are supplied by the recurrent laryngeal nerve (X), except cricothyroid (external branch of the superior laryngeal nerve (X)). The recurrent laryngeal also supplies sensation to the vocal folds and the larynx below them. It lies intimately related to, and often entwined with, branches of the inferior thyroid artery. Great care must be taken to protect this nerve during thyroid surgery. Complete transection of the recurrent laryngeal paralyses the vocal fold, which then lies in a semi-abducted (cadaveric) position. The other fold compensates and speech may be weakened. There is little other effect. Should both nerves be transected, both cords are paralysed and lie in the semiabducted position. Speech, coughing and raising the intra-abdominal pressure become impossible. Should both nerves be bruised or partially injured it is said that the vocal fold adductors take over and the cords adduct to the midline, completely closing the airway, making cricothyroidotomy essential. The superior laryngeal nerve is close to the superior thyroid artery and again care should be taken during surgery. Damage to the external branch paralyses cricothyroid causing some hoarseness of the voice. Damage to the internal branch causes loss of sensation above the vocal folds.

Laryngeal blood supply is by branches of the superior and inferior thyroid arteries and veins. Lymph drains to deep cervical and paratracheal nodes. Laryngeal carcinoma is not uncommon and any alterations to the voice must be investigated.

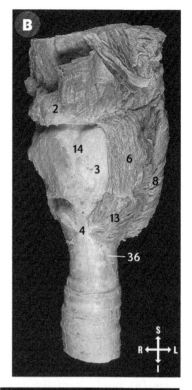

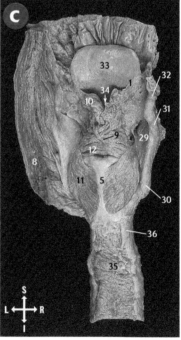

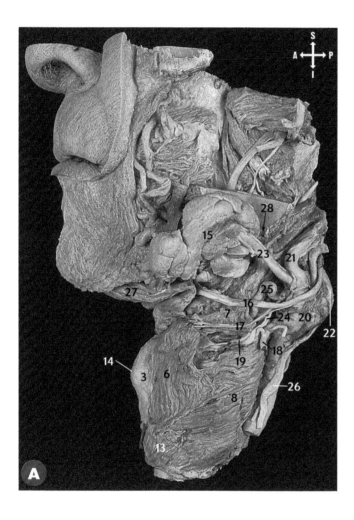

A Side of face, submandibular region and larynx (from the left)
B Larynx (from the front)
C Larynx (from behind)

1	Aryepiglottic fold	11	Posterior crico-arytenoid	20	Bifurcation of common carotid	29	Piriform fossa (recess)

1   Aryepiglottic fold
2   Body of hyoid bone
3   Lamina of thyroid cartilage
4   Arch of cricoid cartilage
5   Lamina of cricoid cartilage
6   Thyrohyoid
7   Stylohyoid
8   Inferior constrictor
9   Oblique arytenoid
10 Aryepiglotticus

11 Posterior crico-arytenoid
12 Transverse arytenoid
13 Cricothyroid
14 Laryngeal prominence
15 Submandibular gland (reflected superiorly)
16 Hypoglossal nerve
17 Nerve to thyrohyoid
18 Superior thyroid artery
19 Superior laryngeal artery

20 Bifurcation of common carotid artery
21 External carotid artery
22 Internal carotid artery
23 Facial artery
24 Internal laryngeal nerve
25 Lingual artery
26 Vagus nerve
27 Anterior belly of digastric
28 Angle of mandible

29 Piriform fossa (recess)
30 Inferior horn of thyroid cartilage
31 Superior horn of thyroid cartilage
32 Greater horn of hyoid bone
33 Epiglottis
34 Vestibule of larynx
35 Trachealis
36 First tracheal cartilage

Location of numbers: 1C; 2B; 3AB; 4B; 5C; 6AB; 7A; 8ABC; 9C; 10C; 11C; 12C; 13AB; 14AB; 15A; 16A; 17A; 18A; 19A; 20A; 21A; 22A; 23A; 24A; 25A; 26A; 27A; 28A; 29C; 30C; 31C; 32C; 33C; 34C; 35C; 36BC.

Superficial anterolateral neck, muscles, fascia

The neck is filled with many important structures that pass between two of three regions: head and neck; upper limb; thorax. The neck is described in triangles. The posterior triangle is between trapezius and sternocleidomastoid, with the clavicle as its base. The anterior triangle is upside down, between sternocleidomastoid and the midline, with the body of the mandible as its base.

Trapezius (1), supplied by the accessory nerve (2), extends the neck, shrugs the shoulders, and helps scapular rotation during abduction of the upper limb. Sternocleidomastoid (3) (accessory nerve) is a prominent feature of the lateral neck. It is related superficially to the external jugular vein (4) and deeply to the internal jugular vein (5) in the carotid neurovascular bundle. The muscle arises by sternal (7) and clavicular (8) heads from the manubrium and from the medial part of the clavicle. These two heads and the intervening fossa may be clearly visible. Sternocleidomastoid attaches to the mastoid process and superior nuchal line on the skull. Acting alone, it laterally flexes the neck to tilt the ear to the ipsilateral shoulder. But it rotates the face in the opposite direc-tion. Such a position (wry neck) may be seen following injury to sternocleidomastoid, or to its nerve supply. Acting together (and with other neck muscles) the two sternocleidomastoids extend the head on the flexed neck, e.g. when straining to look over the heads of a crowd.

The three scalene muscles, anterior, medius (9) and posterior (10), lie in the floor of the posterior triangle. They pass from the cervical transverse processes to the first and second ribs. Consequently, they support the upper thorax during respiration, aiding thoracic elevation in forced inspiration, and they laterally flex the neck. Inferiorly and more deeply, the subclavian artery, surrounded by the trunks of the brachial plexus, emerges between scalenus anterior and scalenus medius.

Levator scapulae (11) passes from the transverse processes of the upper cervical vertebrae to the upper angle of the scapula and helps to elevate and steady the scapula. It is supplied segmentally by cervical ventral rami and by the dorsal scapular nerve. The accessory nerve runs along it in the fascia that forms the roof of the posterior triangle. Splenius capitis (12), arising from the lower cervical and upper thoracic spines, and passing to the mastoid process and superior nuchal line, rotates the head and, as part of erector spinae, is supplied by the upper cervical dorsal rami.

Cervical fascia and spaces

Structures within the neck move in relation to each other, and to the vertebral column, during swallowing and movement of the head. Therefore the structures are surrounded by layers of fascia with potential spaces in between.

The superficial fascia contains subcutaneous fat. Posteriorly the fat is loculated and may be the site of abscesses or carbuncles. Anteriorly it includes platysma muscle. The deep fascia has a series of components. The investing layer of deep fascia forms a supportive collar around the neck. It attaches to the skull, mandible, clavicle and scapular spine, and splits to enclose sternocleidomastoid and trapezius. The prevertebral fascia overlies the anterior vertebral muscles (longus capitis and longus colli) and covers the scalene muscles before fading out laterally over levator scapulae. It passes from the skull base into the thorax, to fuse with the vertebral column at T3–4.

The carotid sheath passes from the skull to the aortic arch and encloses the common and internal carotid arteries, the internal jugular vein and the vagus nerve. It is loose over the vein to allow its distension. The pretracheal fascia passes from the hyoid bone and thyroid cartilage, inferiorly as far as the aortic arch. It splits to enclose the thyroid gland.

The potential spaces between the layers of fascia may form the 'line of least resistance' for the spread of infection, particularly from facial or oral structures. The retropharyngeal space, behind the pharynx and oesophagus extends throughout the neck and posterior thorax from skull to diaphragm. The pretracheal space is in front of the pretracheal fascia and extends from the neck, behind the manubrium to the anterior mediastinum and aortic arch.

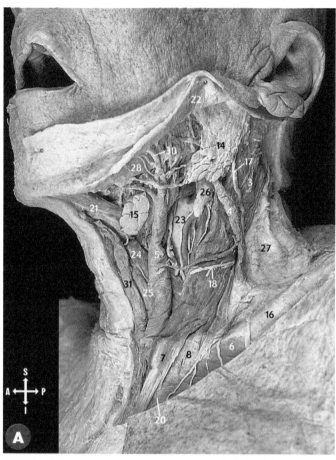

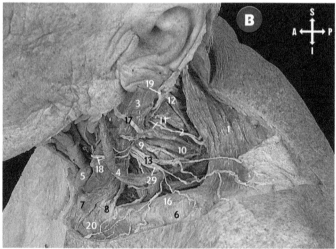

A Anterior triangle of neck (from the front and left)
B Posterior triangle of neck (from the left and above)

1 Trapezius
2 Accessory nerve (spinal part or root)
3 Sternocleidomastoid
4 External jugular vein
5 Interior jugular vein
6 Clavicular part of pectoralis major
7 Sternal head of sternocleidomastoid

8 Clavicular head of sternocleidomastoid
9 Scalenus medius
10 Scalenus posterior
11 Levator scapulae
12 Splenius capitis
13 Cervical nerves to trapezius
14 Parotid gland
15 Submandibular gland (unusually low)

16 Clavicle
17 Great auricular nerve
18 Transverse cervical nerve
19 Lesser occipital nerve
20 Sternocostal part of pectoralis major
21 Anterior belly of digastric
22 Platysma (reflected superiorly)
23 Common carotid artery
24 Omohyoid

25 Sternothyroid
26 Jugulodigastric lymph node
27 Prevertebral fascia
28 Body of mandible
29 Supraclavicular nerves
30 Facial artery
31 Anterior jugular vein

Location of numbers: 1B; 2B; 3AB; 4AB; 5AB; 6AB; 7AB; 8AB; 9B; 10B; 11B; 12B; 13B; 14A; 15A; 16A; 17A; 18AB; 19B; 20AB; 21A; 22A; 23A; 24A; 25A; 26A; 27A; 28A; 29B; 30A; 31A.

Strap muscles, thyroid and parathyroid glands

Strap muscles

The hyoid bone (1) is U-shaped, lies anteriorly in the neck and is palpable just above the thyroid cartilage. It gives origin to muscles that contribute to the pharynx, the tongue and the floor of the mouth. Fine control over the position of the hyoid bone and larynx with consequent control of the position of the tongue, floor of mouth and mandible are essential during speech, swallowing and chewing.

The suprahyoid muscles that connect the hyoid to the mandible (mylohyoid, geniohyoid) and skull are essential to these mechanisms, as are the infrahyoid strap muscles that connect the hyoid bone and thyroid cartilage to the manubrium of the sternum (2) and clavicle (3) (sternohyoid (4), sternothyroid (5)), to the scapula (omohyoid (6)) and to each other (thyrohyoid). The infrahyoid muscles are supplied by the ansa cervicalis, a nerve loop derived from C1–3.

Digastric (8) passes from the mandible to the mastoid process as two bellies connected by an intermediate tendon that passes through a fascial sling attached to the hyoid. The posterior belly is supplied by the facial nerve (cranial nerve VII) and the anterior belly by the nerve to mylohyoid, from the inferior alveolar branch of the third (mandibular) division of the trigeminal nerve (V^3).

With the hyoid held down by the strap muscles inferior to it, digastric is important for pulling the mandible downward to open the mouth. Stylohyoid (VII) is not one of the strap muscles but it lies alongside the posterior belly of digastric and helps control the position of the hyoid.

Thyroid and parathyroid glands

The thyroid gland (Illustration B, 12) lies anteriorly in the lower neck, between the carotid neurovascular bundles, clasping the trachea and the inferior aspect of the larynx. It is a ductless endocrine gland that secretes thyroxin and thyrocalcitonin. The former maintains basal metabolic rate and the correct function and development of many of the body tissues. The latter lowers serum calcium by inhibiting its mobilization from bone.

The shape of the thyroid is variable, but it usually has right and left lobes, united across the second, third and fourth tracheal rings by an isthmus (13). Occasionally a pyramidal lobe extends superiorly from the isthmus. The gland is surrounded by pretracheal fascia that effectively attaches it to the thyroid cartilage. As a result, the thyroid gland moves with the larynx on swallowing. This attachment also prevents the thyroid from enlarging upward; any enlargement must be lateral and inferior, possibly even into the anterior mediastinum.

The parathyroid glands (Illustration C, 15) lie within the thyroid capsule and are variable in number and in position. There are usually four glands, with two each applied to the posterior aspect of each thyroid lobe, one near the upper and one near the lower pole. They secrete parathormone, which mobilizes calcium from the bone to raise serum calcium. Consequently, the parathyroids are necessary for life.

The thyroid and parathyroids are highly vascular and supplied by the superior thyroid branch (16) of the external carotid artery, and the inferior thyroid branch of the subclavian (thyrocervical trunk). There is considerable anastomosis between the left and right arteries and between the superior and inferior arteries. An anastomotic channel between the latter two passes close to the parathyroids and is a landmark for their surgical location. The arteries are related to the laryngeal nerves. Close to the gland the recurrent laryngeal nerve often passes between branches of the inferior thyroid artery. Therefore the inferior thyroid artery must be ligated away from the gland. The superior laryngeal nerve is initially close to the superior thyroid artery but separates from it nearer the gland. Therefore the superior thyroid artery should be ligated close to the gland.

The glands are drained by three veins on each side. The superior and middle veins pass to the internal jugular vein. The inferior thyroid vein (17) may be plexiform and pass to the left brachiocephalic. Lymph drainage is to the deep cervical lymph nodes. Nerve supply is sympathetic, vasomotor, carried on the arteries and derived mainly from the middle cervical ganglion.

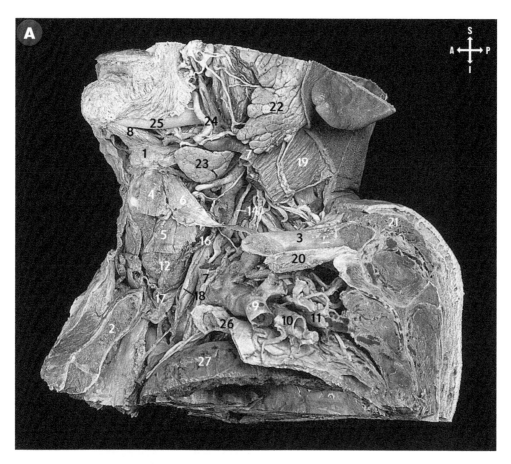

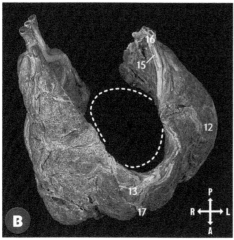

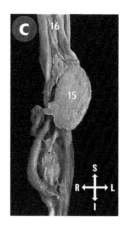

A Neck deep dissection (from the left and slightly below)
B Thyroid gland (from above) with outline of the position
   of the trachea
C Left superior parathyroid gland (from the right)

1	Body of hyoid bone	**8**	Anterior belly of digastric	**15**	Left superior parathyroid gland
2	Manubrium of sternum	**9**	Subclavian vein	**16**	Superior thyroid artery and vein
3	Clavicle	**10**	Subclavian artery	**17**	Inferior thyroid vein
4	Sternohyoid	**11**	Brachial plexus	**18**	Common carotid artery
5	Sternothyroid	**12**	Lateral lobe of thyroid gland	**19**	Sternocleidomastoid
6	Omohyoid	**13**	Isthmus of thyroid gland	**20**	Subclavius
7	Internal jugular vein	**14**	Vagus nerve	**21**	Deltoid

22	Parotid gland
23	Submandibular gland
24	Facial artery and vein
25	Body of mandible
26	First rib
27	Left lung apical lobe

Location of numbers: **1**A; **2**A; **3**A; **4**A; **5**A; **6**A; **7**A; **8**A; **9**A; **10**A; **11**A; **12**AB; **13**B; **14**A; **15**BC; **16**ABC; **17**AB; **18**A; **19**A; **20**A; **21**A; **22**A; **23**A; **24**A; **25**A; **26**A; **27**A.

Deep anterolateral neck, thoracic inlet, arteries, vagus nerves

Deep within the neck, neurovascular structures pass between the neck and the thorax or between the upper limb and the thorax. The first thoracic vertebra, manubrium and first ribs form the thoracic inlet that slopes antero-inferiorly, following the slope of the first rib (1). Scalenus anterior (2) is an important landmark. The apex of each lung (3) extends up to the neck of the first rib. Therefore, the apex is above the anterior end of the first rib, and the medial end of the clavicle (4). Structures in the root of the neck, or thoracic inlet, are related to the apex of the lung and pleura.

The brachiocephalic trunk (5) ascends to the right of the trachea (6) to divide into the right common carotid (7) and the right subclavian (8) artery. On the left the equivalent arteries (9,10) arise directly from the aortic arch.

Subclavian artery and its branches

The subclavian passes upward, medial to the apex of the lung and pleura, then laterally, anterior to the apical pleura and suprapleural membrane (first part), posterior to scalenus anterior (second part) to curve over the first rib (third part) and enter the axilla as the axillary artery (11). It has branches only from the first and second parts. The vertebral artery enters the transverse foramen of the sixth cervical vertebra. It ascends in the transverse foramina, surrounded by a plexus of veins, and a sympathetic plexus from the inferior cervical ganglion, to emerge and pass behind the lateral mass of the atlas to enter the foramen magnum.

The thyrocervical trunk divides into three branches. The transverse cervical and suprascapular arteries pass above the clavicle and across the brachial plexus. They branch to supply the muscles of the neck and also those around the scapula. These latter branches contribute to the scapular anastomosis, which is completed by branches derived from the axillary artery. The inferior thyroid artery (12) takes a tortuous course, deep to the carotid sheath, behind the middle cervical ganglion (from which it picks up sympathetic

fibres) to the lower pole of the thyroid gland, where it is related to the recurrent laryngeal nerve. The inferior thyroid supplies the pharynx and larynx. It also gives off the ascending cervical artery that runs parallel to the phrenic nerve and sends branches to nearby muscles and through the intervertebral foramina to the spinal cord.

The internal thoracic (mammary) artery (13) passes into the thorax to run behind the costal cartilages.

The costocervical trunk divides into two branches: the deep cervical supplies the posterior neck musculature, whereas the highest intercostal descends anterior to the neck of the first rib to provide the posterior intercostal arteries to the first and second spaces.

Carotid arteries

The common carotid arteries lie in the carotid sheath and divide into the external and internal carotid arteries at the upper border of the thyroid cartilage, which is at the lower border of C3 vertebra.

The internal carotid continues upward to enter the skull via the carotid canal and supplies the brain and orbit. The external carotid divides to supply the face, scalp, oral and nasal cavities.

The carotid sinus (a baroreceptor for the control of blood pressure) is a dilatation at the bifurcation of the common carotid, extending to the root of the internal carotid. The carotid body (a chemoreceptor sensitive to low oxygen or high carbon dioxide concentrations in the blood) lies adjacent to the sinus, often wedged between the internal and external carotids. The glossopharyngeal and vagus nerves supply both the sinus and the body.

Vagus nerves

The left and right vagus nerves (X) pass inferiorly in the carotid sheath. Both vagi pass behind the brachiocephalic vein and anterior to the subclavian artery. As the right vagus passes the subclavian it gives the right recurrent laryngeal nerve that then passes behind the carotid artery to the larynx. The left vagus (15) passes with the left carotid and left subclavian to lie on the arch of the aorta. In the neck both vagus nerves give off cardiac branches, as well as pharyngeal and superior laryngeal branches.

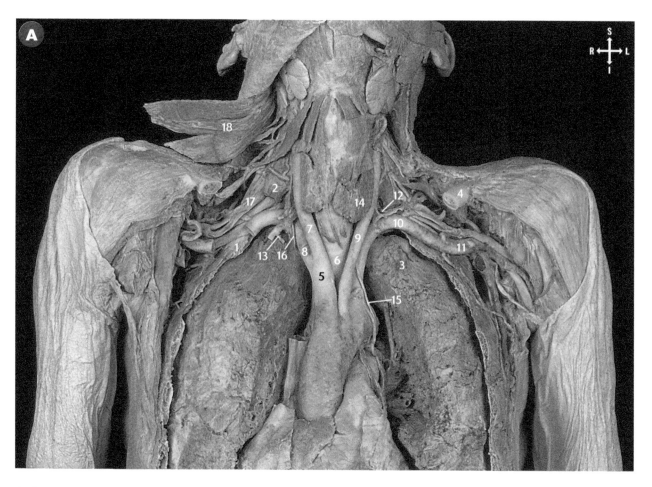

A Deep dissection of the neck and great vessels (from the front)

1	First rib	**6**	Trachea	**12**	Inferior thyroid artery	**17** Brachial plexus
2	Scalenus anterior	**7**	Right common carotid artery	**13**	Internal thoracic (mammary)	**18** Sternocleidomastoid
3	Apex of lung	**8**	Right subclavian artery		artery	
4	Clavicle	**9**	Left common carotid artery	**14**	Lateral lobe of thyroid gland	
5	Brachiocephalic trunk	**10**	Left subclavian artery	**15**	Left vagus nerve	
	(innominate artery)	**11**	Axillary artery	**16**	Right phrenic nerve	

Deep anterolateral neck, veins, nerves

Veins

The jugular venous system drains the head and neck, and is variable.

The external jugular (6) forms opposite the angle of the mandible (or ear lobe) from the posterior auricular vein (draining scalp behind ear) and the posterior branch of the retromandibular vein (formed by the maxillary and superficial temporal veins). It may be visible as it descends superficial to sternocleidomastoid, toward the middle of the clavicle, to enter the subclavian (7) and it has a valve at its termination and one more proximally. It may be used for venous access, but care must be taken to avoid introducing air emboli. Structures in the posterior triangle, the neck, and the scapular muscles usually drain to the external jugular via the variable posterior jugular, suprascapular and transverse cervical veins (11).

Anterior jugulars may be present, one on each side of the midline, superficially. When present, they unite to form the jugular venous arch above the suprasternal notch. The arch passes laterally deep to sternomastoid to enter the external jugular.

The internal jugular (12) receives venous drainage from the intracranial structures (including orbital, nasal and oral cavities), the pharynx, larynx, thyroid gland and face. It lies in the carotid sheath, anterolateral to the internal and then the common carotid artery (13) and commences as the superior jugular bulb in the jugular foramen. It ends at the inferior bulb by joining the subclavian to become the brachiocephalic vein. There is a valve at its termination. The surface marking is from lobe of ear to sternoclavicular joint. A jugular venous pressure wave may be visible just above the clavicle in a patient lying at 45 degrees, particularly in cardiac failure.

The subclavian is the continuation of the axillary vein from the upper limb. It lies parallel to the subclavian artery (14), but more anteriorly and medially, crossing the first rib in front of scalenus anterior (15). The vein may be used for the insertion of central venous lines. Its close proximity to the apex of the pleura and lung makes pneumothorax a common complication of this procedure.

The brachiocephalic vein (internal jugular and subclavian) is formed deep to the sternoclavicular joint. The left vein passes to the right, behind the manubrium and thymus, above the aortic arch, to join the right brachiocephalic and form the superior vena cava deep to the first right costal cartilage. They receive their respective vertebral, internal thoracic, inferior thyroid and highest intercostal veins. The left also receives the left superior intercostal vein, which drains the left second and third intercostal spaces. If the left brachiocephalic lies in a high position it may be at risk during tracheostomy.

Lymph trunks

On the right the jugular, subclavian and mediastinal lymph trunks drain into the right brachiocephalic vein. On the left these trunks usually combine to enter the thoracic duct that enters the junction of the left internal jugular and left subclavian veins. The trunks may enter separately.

Nerves

The sympathetic trunks (17), one on each side, ascend from the thorax to lie on the prevertebral muscles (18), posterior and medial to the carotid artery. Each trunk has a superior ganglion that extends from the skull base to opposite the angle of the mandible, a middle ganglion, and an inferior ganglion that usually fuses with the upper thoracic to lie on the neck of the first rib as the stellate ganglion.

Postganglionic grey rami communicantes leave the ganglia to join the cervical spinal nerves. Other postganglionic branches pass to nearby arteries to be distributed with them. The carotid nerve leaves the superior ganglion to form a plexus on the internal carotid artery. Cardiac branches arise from the cervical sympathetic trunks and descend to supply the heart.

The phrenic nerve (C3,4,5, motor to the diaphragm) passes vertically downward on scalenus anterior, deep to the prevertebral fascia, and slightly lateral to the carotid sheath. Both phrenics pass posterior to the brachiocephalic or subclavian veins. The right stays to the right of the right brachiocephalic vein to run on the superior vena cava. The left phrenic nerve (19) stays lateral to the vagus, the carotid artery and then the aortic arch.

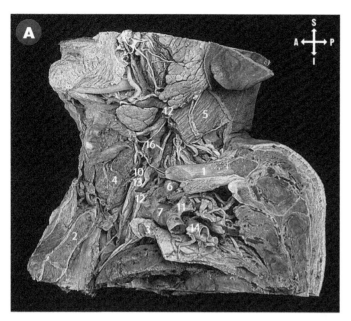

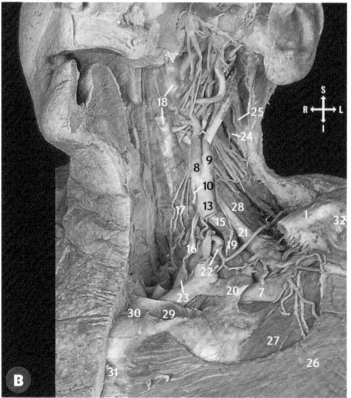

A Neck, deep dissection (from the left and slightly below)

B Neck, deep dissection with pharynx and larynx removed (from the front and left)

1 Clavicle	**11** Suprascapular and transverse cervical veins entering the subclavian vein (a normal variation)	**17** Sympathetic trunk and cardiac branches	**25** Trapezius
2 Manubrium		**18** Prevertebral muscles (longus colli, longus capitis)	**26** Pectoralis major
3 First rib			**27** Pectoralis minor
4 Lateral lobe of thyroid gland	**12** Internal jugular vein	**19** Left phrenic nerve	**28** Scalenus medius
5 Sternocleidomastoid	**13** Common carotid artery	**20** Subclavius	**29** Disc of sternoclavicular joint
6 External jugular vein	**14** Subclavian artery	**21** Upper trunk of brachial plexus	**30** Sternal notch
7 Subclavian vein	**15** Scalenus anterior	**22** Thyrocervical trunk	**31** Body of sternum
8 External carotid artery	**16** Vagus nerve	**23** Vertebral artery	**32** Deltoid
9 Internal carotid artery		**24** Splenius capitis	
10 Superior thyroid artery and vein			

Location of numbers: 1AB; 2A; 3A; 4A; 5A; **6**A; **7**AB; 8B; 9B; 10AB; **11**A; **12**A; **13**AB; **14**A; **15**B; 16AB; **17**B; **18**B; **19**B; 20B; 21B; 22B; 23B; 24B; 25B; 26B; 27B; 28B; 29B; 30B; 31B; 32B.

Part IV

The Thorax

Mediastinum, from left

The organs lying centrally in the thorax comprise the mediastinum, which is divided into four parts: superior, anterior, middle and posterior. The latter three may be grouped as the inferior mediastinum.

Contents

- Superior – great vessels, trachea and oesophagus
- Anterior – thymus and internal thoracic vessels
- Middle – heart and pericardium with the vagus and phrenic nerves
- Posterior – descending aorta, oesophagus, azygos veins and thoracic duct

The thoracic vertebrae and ribs lie posterior to the mediastinum. The manubrium, sternum and the costal cartilages (2) lie anteriorly. The manubriosternal joint is a symphysis of fibrocartilage; it lies opposite T4–T5 and is palpable as the sternal angle of Louis. The superior mediastinum is above T4–5 and behind the manubrium.

The pericardium (3) on the left covers the left ventricle (4), and on the right, the right atrium. Each lung hilum (5–8) is a mirror image of the medial surface of the equivalent lung.

The internal thoracic (mammary) artery (9) sends anterior intercostal arteries into each intercostal space, and is an important blood supply to the breast. It divides into the musculophrenic artery, which supplies the diaphragm, and the superior epigastric artery, which supplies the muscles of the anterior abdominal wall. The internal thoracic may be surgically re-routed to augment or replace occluded coronary arteries. The anastomosis between the superior and inferior epigastrics may open as a collateral circulation.

The thymus lies anteriorly in the mediastinum. In the adult it is largely replaced by fat. But it is important during childhood as a producer of T-lymphocytes, which have immunological function but have been programmed to recognize and not destroy 'self'.

The ascending aorta gives the left and right coronary arteries, then ascends to the right of the trachea, to become the arch of the aorta at T4–5. The aortic arch (10) lies opposite T3 and T4, and has three branches: the brachiocephalic trunk, the left common carotid (11) and the left subclavian (12) arteries. The descending aorta (15) continues from the arch at T4/5, and gives bronchial, oesophageal and posterior intercostal (16) branches. The latter anastomose with the anterior intercostals. The descending aorta lies on the vertebral column, just to the left of the midline, but then moves to the midline to pass behind the diaphragm at T12.

The phrenic and vagus nerves on each side enter the thorax between the subclavian vein and subclavian artery, the vagus being more medial. The courses are then asymmetrical. The left phrenic nerve (18) passes inferiorly, on the pericardium of the left ventricle, before passing through the central tendon of the diaphragm. Both phrenics give motor supply to the diaphragm, as well as sensory supply to the pericardium, mediastinal and diaphragmatic pleura, and peritoneum underlying the diaphragm.

The left vagus (19) runs with the left common carotid to reach the arch of the aorta, which it crosses before giving the recurrent laryngeal nerve (RLN). The left RLN is at risk of compression by tumours and aneurysms at the left lung hilum. The left vagus passes posteriorly, the left phrenic stays anterior, therefore the two nerves cross each other on the aortic arch with the left superior intercostal vein (20) between them. Both vagi pass posterior to the lung hilum. They supply the pulmonary plexuses (bronchoconstriction) and then combine to form an oesophageal plexus, which coalesces to pass through the diaphragm (with the oesophagus) as the anterior (mainly left) and posterior (mainly right) vagal trunks.

The thoracic duct, the main lymph trunk of the body, is the continuation of the abdominal cisterna chyli, and carries lymph from the whole body except the right thorax, right upper limb and right half of the head and neck. It passes behind the diaphragm with the aorta and azygos vein. Aortic pulsation promotes the return flow of both lymph and venous blood. The duct ascends in the midline, or just to the right, until T5, where it crosses to the left, behind the oesophagus. It passes upward in the superior mediastinum and then arches over the apex of the left lung and pleura to enter the formation of the left brachiocephalic vein.

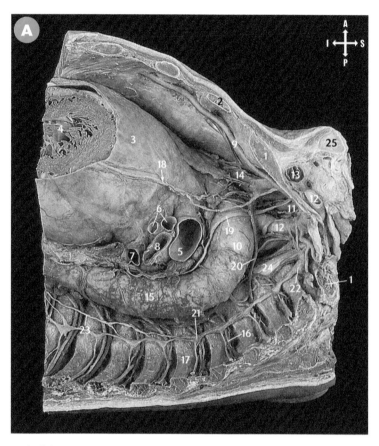

A Left lung root and mediastinum (from the left)

1 First rib	**8** Left main bronchus	**15** Descending thoracic aorta	**22** Cervicothoracic (stellate)
2 Second costal cartilage	**9** Internal thoracic (mammary)	**16** Posterior intercostal artery, vein	ganglion
3 Pericardium	artery and vein	and nerve	**23** Greater splanchnic nerve
4 Left ventricle	**10** Arch of aorta	**17** Sixth rib	**24** Oesophagus
5 Left pulmonary artery	**11** Left common carotid artery	**18** Left phrenic nerve	**25** Clavicle
6 Left superior pulmonary vein	**12** Left subclavian artery	**19** Left vagus nerve	
(divided)	**13** Left subclavian vein	**20** Left superior intercostal vein	
7 Left inferior pulmonary vein	**14** Left brachiocephalic vein	**21** Sympathetic trunk and ganglion	

Mediastinum, from right

The trachea (11) is visible from the right but is overlaid by the aortic arch on the left. It divides into the left and right main bronchi at T4/5, in the concavity of the arch of the aorta, adjacent to the bifurcation of the pulmonary artery (trunk). The right vagus nerve (12) lies on it.

The superior vena cava (13), formed behind the first costal cartilage by the fusion of the right (14) and left (15) brachiocephalic veins, enters the right atrium opposite the third costal cartilage. The inferior vena cava (IVC) pierces the diaphragm and immediately enters the right atrium. The right phrenic nerve (16) lies immediately lateral to the right brachiocephalic vein, superior vena cava and pericardium of the right atrium. It passes through the diaphragm with the IVC at the level of T8.

The azygos vein (17) commences in the abdomen and passes behind the diaphragm to enter the thorax. The posterior intercostal veins drain into the azygos system, which also receives bronchial and oesophageal veins. The azygos lies on the vertebral column before passing superior to the right lung hilum to enter the superior vena cava. On the left, upper and lower hemiazygos veins cross the midline to enter the azygos.

Sympathetic innervation

Primary preganglionic sympathetic nerves emerge from the cord in the ventral roots of T1–L2 spinal nerves, but leave as white rami communicantes to enter the sympathetic trunk, where they usually synapse. The sympathetic trunk (18) lies parallel to the vertebral column, from atlas to coccyx and distributes sympathetic innervation throughout the body. The trunk is studded with ganglia, clusters of cell bodies of the secondary, postganglionic sympathetic nerves.

White rami enter the trunk and synapse in adjacent ganglia or pass up or down the trunk to synapse in distant ganglia. Wherever the synapse, the secondary postganglionic sympathetic nerves leave the trunk either as the grey rami communicantes that join all the spinal nerves or they join blood vessels to be distributed accordingly. The stellate ganglion (20) of the sympathetic trunk lies on the neck of the first rib as it passes into the neck. Tumours at the lung apex may compress the trunk and interrupt sympathetic supply to that side of the head – Horner's syndrome (constricted pupil (myosis), drooping eyelid (ptosis), dry face).

Splanchnic nerves to the intestinal tract are an exception. The primary preganglionic sympathetic nerves pass through the trunk without synapsing. The greater splanchnic (21), the lesser, and the least splanchnic nerves leave their origins in the T5–9, T10–11 and T12 segments of the cord, respectively. Having branched from the appropriate spinal nerves to enter the sympathetic trunks, they leave the trunks and pass into the abdomen. They synapse in ganglia on the aorta, associated with, and distributed with, the arteries to the intestine. These nerves also contain afferent fibres that are important when considering referred pain in the abdomen. The nerves are surgically divided in patients with chronic pain (e.g. chronic pancreatitis).

The oesophagus (22) transports food and fluid from the pharynx to the stomach. It commences at C6 and lies in the midline, immediately anterior to the vertebral column but deep to the trachea and then the left atrium. Inferiorly it lies to the right of the descending aorta, but passes anterior to the aorta (itself moving to the midline) to pierce the diaphragm just to the left of the midline (but through the right crus) at T10, and almost immediately enters the stomach.

The oesophagus is supplied by the recurrent laryngeal and vagus nerves. Arteries are from the inferior thyroid, and the aorta, except the lower end, which is supplied by the left gastric artery. The veins form a rich submucosal anastomosis that drains to the azygos system, or to the portal system via the left gastric vein. Therefore, the oesophagus is an important site of portosystemic venous anastomosis. Lymphatic drainage follows the arteries.

Cricopharyngeus forms a sphincter at the upper end of the oesophagus and only opens during swallowing or vomiting. Occasionally the sphincter does not open quickly enough during vomiting, causing pressure to rise within the oesophagus and tear the mucous membrane. The resultant blood is visible in the vomit (haematemesis).

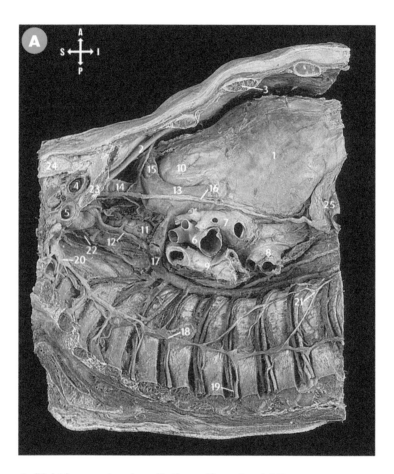

A **Right lung root and mediastinum (from the right)**

1	Pericardium over right atrium	**8**	Inferior right pulmonary vein	**15** Left brachiocephalic vein
2	Internal thoracic (mammary)		(divided)	**16** Right phrenic nerve
	artery and vein	**9**	Right main bronchus (divided)	**17** Azygos vein
3	Third costal cartilage	**10**	Ascending aorta covered by	**18** Sympathetic trunk and ganglion
4	Right subclavian vein		pericardium	**19** Posterior intercostal artery, vein
5	Right subclavian artery	**11**	Trachea	and nerve
6	Right pulmonary artery (divided)	**12**	Right vagus nerve	**20** Cervicothoracic (stellate)
7	Superior right pulmonary vein	**13**	Superior vena cava	ganglion
	(divided)	**14**	Right brachiocephalic vein	**21** Greater splanchnic nerve

22	Oesophagus
23	First rib
24	Clavicle
25	Diaphragm

Thorax: thymus, pleural cavities, thoracic skeleton, intercostal muscles

Pleural cavities

On each side the thoracic cavity appears as if filled with a 'balloon' of serous membrane, the pleura. The parietal layer covers the mediastinum, costal cartilages, ribs and diaphragm. It extends up to the neck of the first rib and down into the costodiaphragmatic recess where the diaphragm attaches inferiorly to the twelfth rib. Each lung invaginates the pleura from its medial side. Therefore, the visceral layer covers the lung and at the hilum (where the vessels and nerves enter and leave) it reflects to become the parietal layer. The visceral pleura dips into the fissures between the lung lobes. The pleural cavity, between the visceral and parietal layers, is a potential space with a minuscule amount of lubricating pleural fluid.

Surface markings

The pleural reflections are mapped on to the thoracic wall in relation to the ribs. The apex is about 2 cm above the medial one-third of the clavicle (2). The pleural cavities lie beside each other in the midline at the level of the second costal cartilage. They continue inferiorly in the midline, but the left deviates to the left at the level of the fourth costal cartilage to make way for the heart, whereas the right cavity continues to the sixth costal cartilage. Laterally, they extend further to reach the eight rib in the midclavicular line, tenth rib in the midaxillary line and twelfth rib posteriorly. The inferior edges of the lungs are two rib spaces higher: the sixth rib in the midclavicular line, eighth rib in the midaxillary line and tenth rib posteriorly.

Ribs, costal cartilages

With the exception of the first, eleventh and twelfth ribs, the head of each rib (3) articulates with its own vertebra, the one above, and the disc between. The tubercle (4) articulates with the transverse process of its own vertebra. Consequently, the neck (5) of each rib slopes downward and laterally. Rib movement is largely by rotation around the axis of that downward-sloping rib neck.

The shaft (6) of each rib also slopes downward as it curves around the chest. The hyaline costal cartilage (7) passes from the end of the rib to the sternum, or to the costal cartilage above, forming the costal margin. The first four costal cartilages are short and horizontal; the others are longer and slope upward. The first rib has a horizontal neck. The eleventh and twelfth ribs have horizontal necks and do not articulate with the sternum or costal margin.

Intercostal muscles

Muscles form three layers within the intercostal spaces. The external intercostal muscle passes downward and forward from one rib to the next, becoming the external intercostal membrane between the costal cartilages. The internal intercostal muscle (8) passes downward and backward from one costal cartilage and rib to the next. It becomes the internal intercostal membrane posteriorly. The innermost layer is incomplete but present anteriorly as transversus thoracis and posteriorly as subcostalis. These innermost muscles cross more than one intercostal space.

The intercostal neurovascular bundle (vein, artery, nerve) lies in the groove inferior to each rib. Their collateral branches runs along the upper border of the rib below. They supply the intercostal muscles, overlying skin and underlying parietal pleura.

Pleural effusion is a collection of excess pleural fluid. Rupture of lung tissue, or of the overlying chest wall, may allow air to enter the pleural cavity (pneumothorax). Associated bleeding will cause a haemopneumothorax. Such collections of air or blood in the pleural cavity are removed by inserting a chest drain into the fifth intercostal space, mid-axillary line. The skin is anaesthetized and incised, and then blunt dissection is used to pass through the intercostal muscles and avoid damage to the neurovascular bundles.

If air enters into the pleural cavity continually, with no route of escape, pressure builds within the cavity to collapse the lung. This is a tension pneumothorax, and the pressure may be high enough to push the heart and trachea off the midline, severely embarrassing respiration and venous return to the heart. The situation is potentially life-threatening, and the pressure must be relieved urgently by a needle in the second intercostal space, midclavicular line.

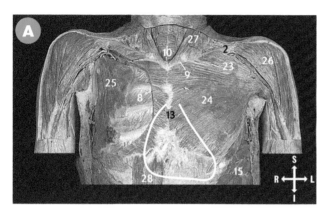

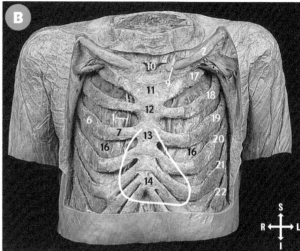

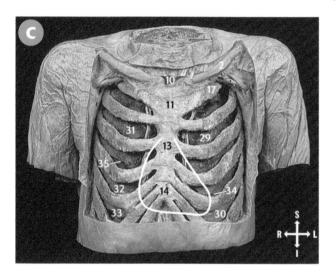

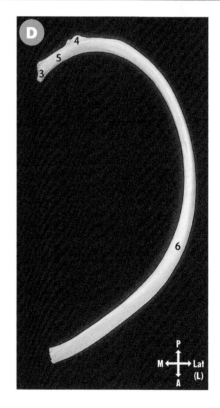

A Muscles of the thoracic wall (from the front)
B Thoracic cavity with ribs, pleural covering and lungs *in situ* (from the front)
C Thoracic cavity with ribs and lungs *in situ* (from the front)
D A left typical rib (from above)

1	Internal thoracic (mammary) artery and vein	**10**	Jugular (suprasternal) notch
2	Clavicle	**11**	Manubrium of sternum
3	Head of rib	**12**	Manubriosternal joint (angle of Louis)
4	Tubercle of rib	**13**	Body of sternum
5	Neck of rib	**14**	Xiphoid process
6	Body (shaft) of rib	**15**	Serratus anterior
7	Costal cartilage	**16**	Pleura over lung
8	Internal intercostal muscle	**17**	First rib
9	Sternoclavicular joint	**18**	Second rib

19	Third rib	**27**	Sternocleidomastoid
20	Fourth rib	**28**	Rectus abdominis
21	Fifth rib	**29**	Superior lobe of left lung
22	Sixth rib	**30**	Inferior lobe of left lung
23	Clavicular part of pectoralis major	**31**	Superior lobe of right lung
24	Sternocostal part of pectoralis major	**32**	Middle lobe of right lung
25	Pectoralis minor	**33**	Inferior lobe of right lung
26	Deltoid	**34**	Oblique fissure of left lung
		35	Transverse fissure of right lung

Location of numbers: 1B; **2**ABC; **3**D; **4**D; **5**D; **6**BD; **7**B; **8**A; **9**AB; **10**ABC; **11**BC; **12**B; **13**ABC; **14**BC; **15**A; **16**B; **17**BC; **18**B; **19**B; **20**B; **21**B; **22**B; **23**A; **24**A; **25**A; **26**A; **27**A; **28**A; **29**C; **30**C; **31**C; **32**C; **33**C; **34**C; **35**C.

Diaphragm

The diaphragm is the primary muscle of inspiration. It arises from the vertebral column, arcuate ligaments, ribs and sternum to form left (1) and right (2) muscular domes that ascend into the thorax and insert into the central tendon (3) of the diaphragm. The nerve supply to each half is by the left and right phrenic (C3,4,5), respectively.

- Diaphragmatic crura – posteriorly a right muscular crus (4) arises from the first three lumbar vertebrae, and a left crus (5) from the first two. The crura both ascend to the central tendon, but the right crus moves to the left to sweep around the lower oesophagus (6) and contribute to its physiological cardiac sphincter.
- Arcuate ligaments – the median arcuate ligament lies at T12 between the two crura. The medial arcuate ligament is formed from the fascia over psoas major (7) and passes from the body to the transverse process of L1. The lateral arcuate ligament is formed from the fascia over quadratus lumborum (8) and runs from the transverse process of L1 to the tip of the twelfth rib. Muscular fibres ascend from the arcuate ligaments to the central tendon. Should the fibres that arise from the medial or lateral ligaments be absent at birth, the abdominal contents will move into the thorax – congenital diaphragmatic hernia (hernias of Bochdalek and Morgagni).

The remaining diaphragm muscle arises from the inner aspects of the lower six ribs and costal cartilages (interdigitating with transversus abdominis) around to the xiphisternum, which also sends muscle fibres to the central tendon.

Structures passing through (or behind) the diaphragm

The aorta (9), thoracic duct (10) and azygos vein (11) pass behind the median arcuate ligament. The oesophagus and the two vagal trunks pass through the right crus, just to the left of the midline at T10.

The splanchnic nerves pierce the crura on their way to the coeliac plexus, which forms around the coeliac

trunk (12). The coeliac trunk arises from the aorta between the crura. The sympathetic chain passes behind the medial arcuate ligament, and the subcostal neurovascular bundle behind the lateral.

The inferior vena cava (13) and right phrenic nerve pass through the central tendon at T8, i.e. behind the right sixth costal cartilage, just to the right of the midline. The left phrenic nerve sends its branches through the left diaphragmatic dome.

Relations

The underlying abdominal relations differ on each side and may be in danger during the insertion of a chest drain or following rib fracture. The liver (14) is on the right, the stomach (16) and spleen (18) on the left. On each side, the kidney (19,20) lies posteriorly in the abdomen, partially on the diaphragm and therefore related to the costodiaphragmatic recess (21).

Diaphragmatic movements

On inspiration the domes flatten to increase the vertical thoracic diameter. With increased respiratory effort the central tendon descends too. But its descent is limited by its attachment to the pericardium (22) and by the underlying abdominal viscera. Further diaphragmatic contraction, in forced inspiration, pulls on the ribs and costal cartilages to evert the seventh to tenth ribs. This 'bucket handle' movement increases the lateral thoracic diameter.

Expiration is by relaxation, elastic recoil and by pressure from the underlying abdominal viscera. The latter may be increased by contraction of the abdominal wall muscles.

The pleura superior to the diaphragm, and the peritoneum inferior to it, both have sensory supply by the phrenic nerve (C3,4,5). Irritation of the undersurface of the diaphragm (cholecystitis, blood from a ruptured spleen) may refer pain to the respective shoulder tip, supplied by C3,4 via the lateral supraclavicular nerve.

Paralysis of one side of the diaphragm will result in paradoxical movement. During inspiration the paralysed side is forced upward (instead of the expected downward movement) by the raised intra-abdominal pressure that is created by descent of the healthy half of the diaphragm.

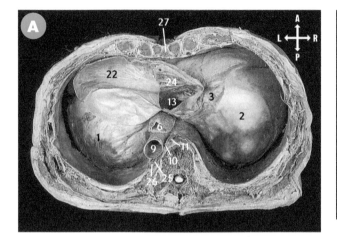

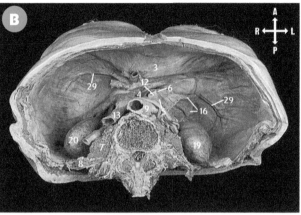

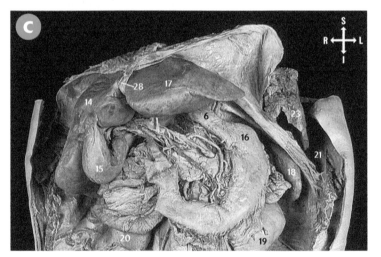

A Diaphragm (from above)
B Diaphragm (from below)
C Upper abdomen, contents (from the front)

1	Left dome of diaphragm	9	Aorta	
2	Right dome of diaphragm	10	Thoracic duct	
3	Central tendon of diaphragm	11	Azygos vein	
4	Right crus of diaphragm	12	Coeliac trunk	
5	Left crus of diaphragm	13	Inferior vena cava	
6	Oesophagus	14	Right lobe of liver	
7	Psoas major	15	Gall bladder	
8	Quadratus lumborum	16	Fundus of stomach	

17	Left lobe of liver
18	Spleen
19	Left kidney
20	Right kidney
21	Costodiaphragmatic recess
22	Fibrous pericardium
23	Lower lobe left lung
24	Right atrium

25	Hemi-azygos vein
26	Left greater splanchnic nerve
27	Body (lower end) of sternum
28	Falciform ligament
29	Inferior phrenic vessels

Location of numbers: 1A; 2A; 3AB; 4B; 5B; 6ABC; 7B; 8B; 9AB; 10A; 11A; 12B; 13AB; 14C; 15C; 16BC; 17C; 18C; 19BC; 20BC; 21C; 22A; 23C; 24A; 25A; 26A; 27A; 28C; 29B.

Lungs: lobes, fissures, bronchi, hila, relations

The lungs are for respiration, the exchange of oxygen and carbon dioxide between the blood and the atmosphere. Respiration ensures oxygenation of the blood and also maintains its correct pH.

Lung surface projections are the same as the pleura, except inferiorly where they are two rib spaces higher (p. 68). On full or forced inspiration the lungs descend into the costodiaphragmatic recesses.

Lobes and fissures

Both lungs are divided into an upper and a lower lobe by the oblique fissure (1). The transverse fissure (2) further subdivides the right upper lobe. So the left lung has two lobes (3,4) and the right lung three lobes (5,6,7). Surface projection of each oblique fissure is to the spines of T3/T4 (palpable on examination) or the body of T5 (visible on a radiograph) and then around the chest to the sixth rib. The transverse fissure is deep to the right fourth costal cartilage and rib, meeting the oblique fissure at the fifth rib. Surface projection of the fissures allows approximate location of the lung lobes and segments during examination of the thorax. Essentially, the upper lobe is anterior, the lower lobe posterior, and the middle lobe lateral.

Bronchi and bronchopulmonary segments

The trachea and bronchi are fibro-elastic tubes, held open by cartilage, but with muscle in their walls to control diameter. The muscle contracts under parasympathetic stimulation in quiet respiration, reducing the dead space. The muscle relaxes, under sympathetic control, to allow increased airflow as respiratory demand rises. Asthma is the excessive constriction of the bronchioles. One therapy uses drugs that have a sympathetic effect of dilating the bronchi.

The right main bronchus (8) is shorter, wider and more vertical than the left, therefore more likely to receive foreign bodies. The left lung is displaced to the left by the heart, so looks longer and narrower than the right lung, but this also means that the left bronchus (9) is longer and more horizontal.

Within the lung, or just outside it, the bronchi divide into lobar (secondary bronchi) and then bron-chopulmonary segments (tertiary bronchi). These segments may be surgically removed or be the location of a pneumonia. Each upper lobe has an apical, an anterior and a posterior segment. Each lower lobe has an apical segment and four basal segments, medial, lateral, anterior and posterior. The middle lobe (6) on the right has medial and lateral segments. The lingula (10) is the equivalent on the left, with upper and lower segments. On each side, there are ten segments in all, but the heart causes some on the left to be small.

The first tertiary bronchus to arise from the bronchial tree posteriorly is to the apical segment of the lower lobe (11), which is therefore prone to pneumonia. It lies high in the thorax adjacent to the T4 spine.

The hilum contains lymph nodes, and bronchial arteries and veins to supply the bronchi and lung tissue. The bronchial arteries arise from the aorta or posterior intercostal arteries. The bronchial veins drain to the azygos system. Each hilum receives air via its bronchus, and de-oxygenated blood via its pulmonary artery. The left bronchus and the left pulmonary artery (12) are single. But the right bronchus and the right pulmonary artery (13) bifurcate just before the hilum so the right hilum has two bronchi and two arteries. Both hila have two main (superior (14) and inferior (15)) pulmonary veins to carry oxygenated blood back to the left atrium. The bronchi tend to be posterior, the pulmonary arteries anterosuperior, and the pulmonary veins antero-inferior.

Lymph drainage

The lung is drained by plexuses of lymph vessels that lie on the bronchi and under the pleura. They converge on the hilar lymph nodes (16), which send afferents to the tracheobronchial nodes and then to the mediastinal nodes. Lung tumour may spread to these nodes and be seen on radiographs as a slight widening of the mediastinum.

Relations

Apart from the phrenic and vagus nerves, the mediastinal relations are different for each lung. The left is related to the left ventricle, aortic arch, descending aorta and oesophagus inferiorly. The right lung is related to the superior vena cava, trachea, azygos vein and right atrium.

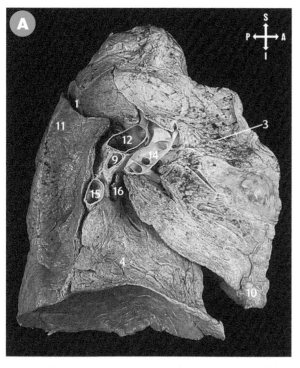

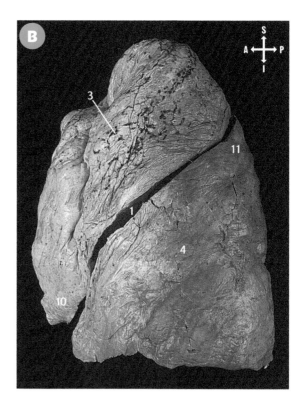

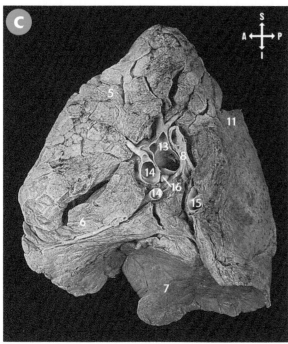

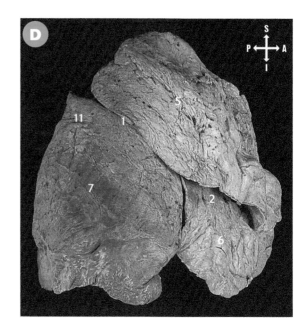

A Left lung, medial aspect (from the right)
B Left lung, lateral aspect (from the left)
C Right lung, medial aspect (from the left)
D Right lung, lateral aspect (from the right)

1	Oblique fissure	5	Superior lobe of right lung	9	Left main bronchus	13	Right pulmonary artery (divided)
2	Transverse fissure	6	Middle lobe of right lung	10	Lingula of left lung	14	Superior pulmonary veins (divided)
3	Superior lobe of left lung	7	Inferior lobe of right lung	11	Apical segment of lower lobe	15	Inferior pulmonary veins
4	Inferior lobe of left lung	8	Right main bronchus (divided)	12	Left pulmonary artery	16	Hilar lymph nodes

Location of numbers: 1ABD; 2D; 3AB; 4AB; 5CD; 6CD; 7CD; 8C; 9A; 10AB; 11ABCD; 12A; 13C; 14AC; 15AC; 16AC.

Heart: *in situ* and removed

The heart lies centrally within the thorax and is the muscular pump that receives, on its right side, de-oxygenated blood, which is pumped to the lungs for oxygenation. The oxygenated blood returns from the lungs to the left side of the heart to be pumped into the systemic circulation. Consequently, there are right and left receiving chambers, the atria, and right and left pumping chambers, the ventricles.

Pericardium

The heart is enclosed in the pericardial sac (1) in the middle mediastinum. The external layer of fibrous pericardium is lined by serous parietal pericardium. Where the major vessels pierce the pericardium to enter or leave the heart, the parietal layer reflects onto the vessels and continues around the heart as the visceral pericardium (epicardium). The resultant, lubricated potential space between the parietal and visceral layers allows cardiac movement and contraction.

Within the pericardial sac, between the visceral and parietal layers there are the oblique and transverse sinuses. The former is a potential space behind the left atrium (2) to allow its expansion. The latter has the ascending aorta (3) and pulmonary trunk (4) anteriorly, the superior vena cava (5) and the upper aspect of the left atrium posteriorly. During cardiac surgery slings and clamps are passed through the transverse sinus to control blood flow in the great vessels.

The fibrous pericardium fuses with the great vessels superiorly and the central tendon of the diaphragm (10) inferiorly. This latter attachment limits the descent of the central tendon.

Nerve supply and referred pain

The fibrous and parietal pericardia both receive sensation via the phrenic nerves. The visceral pericardium, like the heart itself, receives sensation via the sympathetics. Although the cardiac branches descend into the thorax from the cervical parts of the sympathetic trunks, their origin in the spinal cord is from T1–5 segments. Therefore pain from the heart and visceral pericardium usually refers to the anterior chest wall. But it may also extend into the T1 and T2 dermatomes down the inner aspect of the left arm. Blood and fluid may collect within the pericardial sac, which can reduce venous return and cardiac contraction – cardiac tamponade.

The heart lies behind the sternum but extends to the left. In the sagittal plane it lies obliquely so that the apex (12) is anterior and the base posterior. The right border is the right atrium (13). The anterior (sternocostal) surface is mainly right ventricle (14). The left border and apex is left ventricle. The inferior surface lies on the diaphragm and is formed mainly by left ventricle and partially right ventricle. The base, which is left atrium, lies posteriorly, related to the oesophagus and descending aorta opposite T5–7.

Surface projections of the four corners of the heart (Illustration B)

- Upper left – at the left second costal cartilage, parasternally (P)
- Upper right – at the right third costal cartilage parasternally (A)
- Lower right – at the right sixth costal cartilage, parasternally (or T8 where the inferior vena cava pierces the diaphragm and immediately enters the right atrium) (T)
- Lower left – or apex (palpable) at the left fifth intercostal space, mid-clavicular line (M)

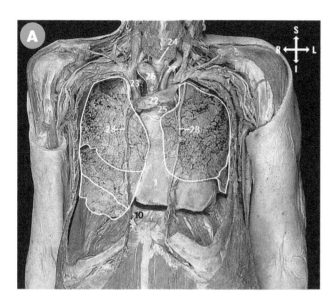

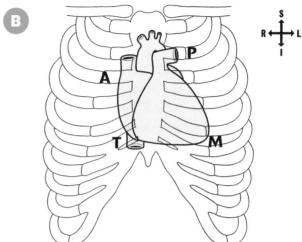

Surface projections of the four corners of the heart

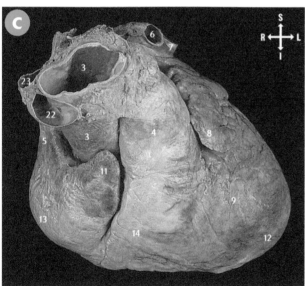

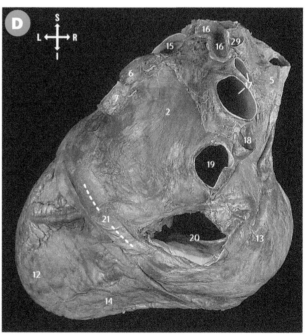

A Thorax with ribcage removed (from the front)
B Ribs and heart, surface markings (from the front)
C Heart (from the front)
D Heart (from behind)

1	Pericardium	9	Left ventricle	17	Right pulmonary artery (divided)
2	Left atrium	10	Central tendon of diaphragm	18	Right superior pulmonary vein
3	Ascending aorta	11	Right auricle	19	Right inferior pulmonary vein
4	Pulmonary artery (trunk)	12	Apex of heart	20	Inferior vena cava
5	Superior vena cava	13	Right atrium	21	Coronary sinus in atrioventricular
6	Left superior pulmonary vein	14	Right ventricle		(coronary) groove
7	Left inferior pulmonary vein	15	Left pulmonary artery	22	Left brachiocephalic vein
8	Left auricle	16	Left and right main bronchi	23	Right brachiocephalic vein

24 Trachea
25 Arch of aorta
26 Brachiocephalic trunk
27 Left common carotid artery
28 Internal thoracic (mammary)
    artery
29 Azygos vein

Location of numbers: 1A; 2D; 3C; 4C; 5CD 6CD; 7CD; 8C; 9C; 10A; 11C; 12CD; 13CD; 14CD; 15D; 16D; 17D; 18D; 19D; 20D; 21D; 22AC; 23AC; 24A; 25A; 26A; 27A; 28A; 29D.

Heart: chambers

During the cardiac cycle blood is ejected from the ventricles by their contraction during systole. During diastole the ventricles relax and are filled with blood by atrial contraction. The atrioventricular valves ensure unidirectional flow from atrium to ventricle.

The interventricular septum (1) separates the left (2) and right (3) ventricles. On the surface, that separation is visible anteriorly and posteriorly as the interventricular groove (4). Similarly, on both surfaces the atrioventricular groove, between the two atria and the two ventricles, is visible and represents the position of the figure-of-eight fibrous skeleton that separates the atria from the ventricles. The fibrous skeleton lies obliquely, just off the coronal plane. It houses the atrioventricular valves and it breaks the wave of con- duction from the atria to the ventricles. Congenital and pathologically acquired defects can occur in the interventricular septum allowing the shunting of blood from the left to the right side of the heart (ventricular septal defect or VSD).

The interatrial septum (5) separates the right atrium from the left atrium. As the right atrium is actually anterior to the left, the septum forms the posterior wall of the right atrium. Both atria develop from original fetal atrium, and also from the incorporation of original fetal vein. The auricles, ridged by musculi pectinati are the remnants of fetal atrium, whereas the smooth part of each atrium represents fetal vein. The right atrium (6) receives both the superior (7) and inferior vena cavae (8) and the coronary sinus (9). The crista terminalis (10) is an internal ridge running longitudinally between the vena cavae. Musculi pectinati (11) run from the crista terminalis into the auricle (12).

The interatrial septum, lying posteriorly, shows the fossa ovalis (13), which indicates the position of the fetal foramen ovale. In the fetus, blood bypasses the pulmonary circulation by flowing through the foramen ovale from right to left atrium. The foramen closes at birth, but many people have asymptomatic 'probe patency'. That is, after death, a probe may be passed through a residual aperture in the interatrial septum.

During diastole blood passes through the tricuspid valve (14) into the right ventricle, which appears crescent-shaped and wraps around the thicker, circular left ventricle. The right ventricle has muscular ridges, trabeculae carneae (20) that smooth out and disappear towards the infundibulum, which leads to the pulmonary trunk.

The atrial and ventricular muscular ridges give power of contraction, without taking up space or making the heart walls excessively thick. Their disappearance and return to a smooth surface ensures laminar blood flow.

The left atrium (21) is quadrangular and on the base of the heart, posteriorly. It has an auricle but is mainly smooth and receives oxygenated blood via the left (27) and right (28) superior and inferior pulmonary veins. During diastole blood passes through the bicuspid mitral valve to the left ventricle. The left ventricle has numerous fine trabeculae carneae, which decrease towards the aortic vestibule, to ensure laminar flow.

In both ventricles there are papillary muscles associated with valve function.

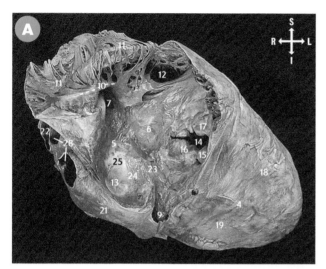

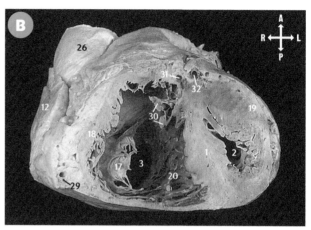

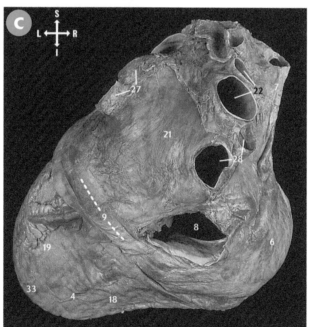

A Open right atrium (from the front and right)
B Axial section through the ventricles (from below)
C Heart (from behind)

1	Muscular part of interventricular septum	10	Crista terminalis
2	Left ventricle	11	Musculi pectinati
3	Right ventricle	12	Right auricle
4	Position of interventricular groove (posteriorly)	13	Fossa ovalis
5	Interatrial septum	14	Tricuspid valve
6	Right atrium	15	Posterior cusp of tricuspid valve
7	Superior vena cava	16	Septal cusp of tricuspid valve
8	Inferior vena cava	17	Anterior cusp of tricuspid valve
9	Coronary sinus	18	Right ventricular wall
		19	Left ventricular wall
20	Trabeculae carneae in right ventricle	29	Marginal branch of right coronary artery
21	Left atrium	30	Septal papillary muscle
22	Right pulmonary artery	31	Anterior interventricular (descending) branch of left coronary artery in interventricular groove
23	Position of atrioventricular node		
24	Limbus fossa ovalis		
25	Position of intravenous tubercle of interatrial septum	32	Great cardiac vein
26	Ascending aorta	33	Apex of heart
27	Left pulmonary veins		
28	Right pulmonary veins		

Location of numbers: 1B; 2B; 3B; 4AC; 5A; 6AC; 7AC; 8C; 9AC; 10A; 11A; 12AB; 13A; 14A; 15A; 16A; 17AB; 18ABC; 19ABC; 20B; 21AC; 22AC; 23A; 24A; 25A; 26B; 27C; 28AC; 29B; 30B; 31B; 32B; 33C.

Heart valves and conducting system

The atrioventricular valves are both opened and closed by the pressure of blood. Flow of blood during atrial contraction (diastole) pushes the cusps into the ventricle. During ventricular contraction (systole) the blood pressure pushes the valves shut and the papillary muscles and chordae tendineae prevent the cusps from everting into the atrium.

The tricuspid valve (1) has posterior (or inferior) (2), septal (3) and anterior (4) cusps. There are respective papillary muscles (5,6), but each of these sends chordae tendineae (7) to two cusps. Consequently, the cusps are drawn together as well as being held shut.

The mitral valve has two cusps, the anterior (8) and posterior (9) cusps. There are equivalent papillary muscles (10,11), although each sends chordae tendineae to both cusps. The anterior cusp is smooth on both surfaces as it lies between the ventricular inflow and its outflow, the aortic vestibule.

Auscultation

The atrioventricular and arterial valves lie in a line – pulmonary, aortic, mitral and tricuspid – behind the sternum. On auscultation their sounds are best heard by following the direction in which blood flows as it passes through each valve:

- Tricuspid – sixth right interspace or at the lower end of the sternum
- Mitral – at cardiac apex, left fifth interspace, midclavicular line
- Aortic – right second intercostal space
- Pulmonary – left second intercostal space

The valves may be diseased and become narrowed (stenosed) or leak (incompetent). Additional abnormal murmurs are heard on auscultation during the cardiac cycle.

The cardiac conducting system

The heart must beat continually and rhythmically. Heart rate is slowed by parasympathetic supply from the cervical parts of the vagus nerves and their recurrent laryngeal branches. Heart rate is raised by sympathetic supply that reaches the heart in branches descending from the cervical parts of the left and right sympathetic trunks. The parasympathetic and sympathetic branches converge on superficial and deep cardiac plexuses that lie together at the ligamentum arteriosum and bifurcations of the pulmonary trunk and trachea. These three points are immediately adjacent to each other. The plexuses send branches into the heart with the coronary arteries. They also supply the sinu-atrial node, or pacemaker of the heart.

The sinu-atrial node (24) lies at the upper end of the crista terminalis (25), which is just at the entry of the superior vena cave (26), where the auricle joins the atrium. Conduction and consequent contraction spread through the atria to propel blood toward and through the atrioventricular valves.

The conduction must not continue, unco-ordinated, straight into the ventricles. If it did so, the contraction may be not only irregular but also in the wrong direction, toward the inferior end of each ventricle. Consequently, the atrioventricular node (27), in the inferior aspect of the interatrial septum, 'gathers' the conduction and transmits it through the cardiac fibrous skeleton and into the bundle of His.

The bundle of His passes down the interventricular septum (34), to divide into right and left bundles that branch out into each ventricle. The wave of conduction and contraction is then synchronous, and from the lower aspect of each ventricle up toward its outflow. In the right ventricle the moderator band (septomarginal trabeculum) carries conduction from the right branch of the bundle of His to the base of the anterior papillary muscle. This ensures it is ready to contract in synchrony with the other papillary muscles

Abnormalities of cardiac rhythm severely affect cardiac function. Excessive ventricular tachycardia or fibrillation renders cardiac function as useless as if the heart had stopped beating altogether. Both conditions can result in cardiac arrest. The coronary arteries fill during diastole. Abnormal rhythm may prevent normal coronary artery filling and cause cardiac ischaemia.

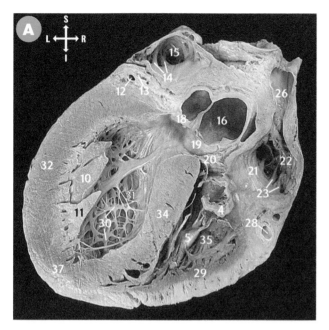

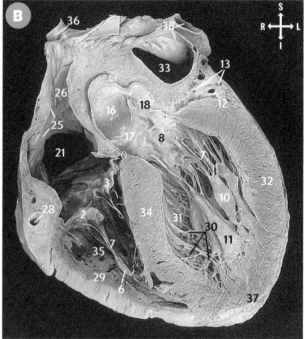

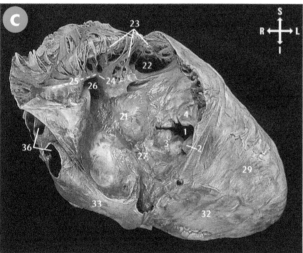

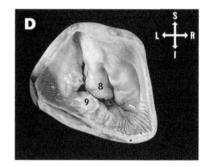

A Heart, coronal section – anterior portion (from behind)
B Heart, coronal section – posterior portion (from the front)
C Opened right atrium (from the front and right)
D Closed mitral valve (from behind)

1	Tricuspid valve	10	Anterior papillary muscle of left ventricle
2	Posterior cusp of tricuspid valve	11	Posterior papillary muscle of left ventricle
3	Septal cusp of tricuspid valve	12	Great cardiac vein
4	Anterior cusp of tricuspid valve	13	Left coronary artery branches
5	Anterior papillary muscle of right ventricle	14	Musculi pectinati in left auricle
6	Posterior papillary muscle of right ventricle	15	Left auricle
7	Chordae tendineae	16	Ascending aorta
8	Anterior cusp of mitral valve	17	Posterior cusp of aortic valve
9	Posterior cusp of mitral valve	18	Left cusp of aortic valve
		19	Right cusp of aortic valve

20	Membranous part of interventricular septum
21	Right atrium
22	Right auricle
23	Musculi pectinati in right auricle
24	Position of sinu-atrial node
25	Crista terminalis
26	Superior vena cava
27	Position of atrioventricular node
28	Right coronary artery in atrioventricular groove
29	Right ventricular wall

30	Trabeculae carneae in left ventricle
31	Left ventricle
32	Left ventricular wall
33	Left atrium
34	Interventricular septum
35	Right ventricle
36	Right pulmonary veins
37	Apex of heart
38	Left pulmonary veins entering left atrium

Location of numbers: 1C; 2BC; 3BC; 4AC; 5A; 6B; 7B; 8BD; 9D; 10AB; 11AB; 12AB 13AB; 14A; 15A; 16AB; 17B; 18AB; 19A; 20AB; 21ABC; 22AC; 23AC; 24C; 25BC; 26ABC; 27C; 28AB; 29ABC; 30AB; 31AB; 32ABC; 33BC; 34AB; 35AB; 36BC; 37AB; 38B.

Heart: superior and external views, major vessels, coronary arteries and veins

Superior aspect of the heart

The superior vena cava (1), which carries de-oxygenated blood from the head, neck, upper limbs and thoracic wall, enters the right atrium. The pulmonary trunk (2) leaves the right ventricle and divides into the left (3) and right (4) pulmonary arteries that carry de-oxygenated blood to each lung.

The aorta (5) leaves the left ventricle, ascends and then arches backward over the pulmonary trunk and left main bronchus (6), before becoming the descending aorta at T4/5. It distributes oxygenated (arterial) blood to the systemic (body) circulation. As it emerges from the heart the aorta is slightly posterior and to the right of the pulmonary trunk, between it and the superior vena cava.

The right (8) and left (9) auricles extend from their respective atria around the base of the aorta and pulmonary trunk.

Aortic and pulmonary valves

Blood is ejected from the ventricles by their contraction during systole. The aorta and pulmonary trunk are elastic arteries and their elastic recoil during diastole propels blood onward.

The pulmonary (14,15,16) and aortic (17,18,19) valves all have three semilunar cusps that are forced outward against the wall of each vessel during systole. Above each cusp there is a small dilation or sinus. During diastole, the elastic recoil not only forces blood onward but also creates back pressure, which forces blood into the sinuses between the cusps and the vessel wall. Therefore the cusps are forced to meet each other in the middle of the arterial lumen to occlude it and prevent backflow into the ventricles.

Various diseases may cause the valves to become narrowed (stenosis), and/or allow leakage of blood back into the ventricle during diastole (incompetent).

Cardiac blood supply

The coronary arteries arise from two of the sinuses in the ascending aorta. The right coronary artery (20) emerges from the sinus above the right cusp. It lies in the atrioventricular groove and passes to the inferior border of the heart. It gives the marginal artery (21) before continuing on the postero-inferior surface, in the atrioventricular groove, to give the posterior interventricular artery (22) in the posterior interventricular groove.

The left coronary artery (23) arises from the sinus above the left cusp. It divides into the circumflex artery (24), which continues around the heart in the atrioventricular groove, and the anterior interventricular (25) (left anterior descending), which lies in the groove of the same name.

The right coronary usually supplies the sino-atrial node (sixty per cent) and the atrioventricular node (ninety per cent). Branches of the coronary arteries do anastomose with each other, but not effectively enough to prevent myocardial ischaemia or infarction. The anterior and posterior interventricular arteries send branches into the interventricular septum to supply the conductive bundle of His and its branches. Arterial occlusion and consequent infarction may cause abnormalities of cardiac rhythm. The posterior interventricular usually comes from the right coronary – right cardiac dominance. But it may be a continuation of the anterior interventricular, from the left coronary – left cardiac dominance. Narrowed (stenosed) coronary arteries, resulting in cardiac ischaemia, can be dilated with balloon angioplasty and metallic stents. Occluded coronary arteries may be surgically bypassed using grafts from the great saphenous vein, or from the internal thoracic artery.

The great cardiac vein (26) lies in the anterior interventricular groove, but curves (with the circumflex artery) onto the posterior surface in the atrioventricular groove. It becomes the coronary sinus (27) that runs along the inferior surface of the left atrium to open into the right atrium. Most cardiac veins are tributaries of the coronary sinus. But the anterior cardiac vein drains the wall of the right ventricle into the right atrium. Many tiny veins are found within the cardiac muscle, particularly on the right side. These are venae cordis minimae, and these drain directly into the chambers.

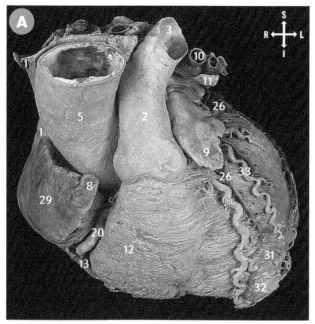

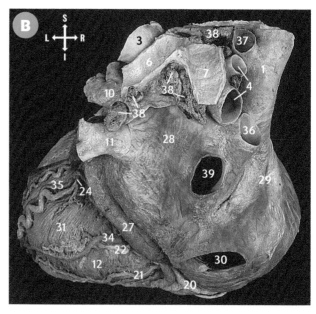

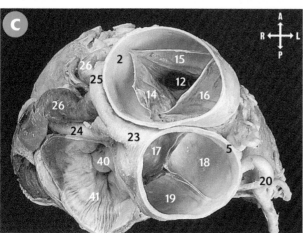

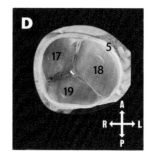

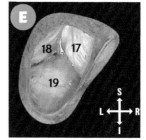

A   Heart, dissected (from the front)
B   Heart, dissected (from behind)
C   Pulmonary valve (open), aortic valve (closed) and mitral valve (closed) (from behind)

D   Aortic valve (closed) (from above)
E   Aortic valve (closed) (from below)

1	Superior vena cava	15	Left cusp of open pulmonary valve
2	Pulmonary trunk	16	Right cusp of open pulmonary valve
3	Left pulmonary artery	17	Left cusp of closed aortic valve
4	Right pulmonary arteries	18	Right cusp of closed aortic valve
5	Ascending aorta	19	Posterior (non-coronary) cusp of closed aortic valve
6	Left main bronchus	20	Right coronary artery in atrioventricular groove
7	Right main bronchus	21	Right marginal artery
8	Right auricle	22	Posterior interventricular artery in interventricular groove
9	Left auricle	23	Left coronary artery
10	Superior left pulmonary vein	24	Circumflex branch of left coronary artery
11	Inferior left pulmonary vein	25	Anterior interventricular branch of left coronary artery, in interventricular groove
12	Right ventricle	26	Great cardiac vein
13	Small cardiac vein	27	Coronary sinus in atrioventricular (coronary) groove
14	Posterior cusp of open pulmonary valve	28	Left atrium
		29	Right atrium
		30	Inferior vena cava
		31	Left ventricle
		32	Apex of heart
		33	Left marginal artery

34   Middle cardiac vein in posterior interventricular groove
35   Left posterior ventricular vein
36   Superior right pulmonary vein
37   Azygos vein
38   Tracheobronchial lymph nodes
39   Inferior right pulmonary vein
40   Anterior cusp of closed mitral valve
41   Posterior cusp of closed mitral valve

Location of numbers: 1AB; 2AC; 3AB; 4B; 5ACD; 6B; 7B; 8A; 9A; 10AB; 11AB; 12ABC; 13A; 14C; 15C; 16C; 17CDE; 18CDE; 19CDE; 20ABC; 21B; 22B; 23C; 24BC; 25AC; 26AC; 27B; 28B; 29AB; 30B; 31AB; 32A; 33A; 34B; 35B; 36B; 37B; 38B; 39B; 40C; 41C.

The breast, and the thoracic wall in respiration

Breast

The breast, for nutrition of the newborn, is a modified sweat gland, with fifteen to twenty lobes embedded in fat (1), emptying into lactiferous ducts (2) and via ampullae under the areola (3) into the nipple (4). During pregnancy the lobes enlarge (like bunches of grapes). Males have rudimentary breast tissue.

The breast lies on the second to sixth ribs in the midclavicular line, on the deep fascia overlying pectoralis major (5), serratus anterior (6), and the upper end of external oblique (7). An axillary tail may curve under pectoralis major, pierce the deep fascia and enter the axilla. The submammary space, between the deep fascia and the breast, allows it some movement in relation to the underlying muscle. Suspensory ligaments (8) between the deep fascia and breast dermis support the breast. These may shorten with tumour involvement and cause skin puckering. Similarly, advanced tumour may invade the submammary space and anchor the breast.

The position of the nipple and areola varies but usually they are at the level of the fourth intercostal space in the young female. They are pink (depending on race) in the nulliparous female, but darken to pale brown after pregnancy. The areola has many sebaceous glands, which have a lubricating, protective function during suckling.

Branches of the internal thoracic and anterior intercostal arteries (especially the third and fourth) supply the breast medially, and superior thoracic, thoracoacromial and lateral thoracic (9) branches of axillary artery laterally. The arteries have equivalent veins. Lymph drainage usually follows the arteries. Medially it is to parasternal nodes alongside the internal thoracic artery. Most lymph, seventy-five per cent, passes laterally to the nodes of the axilla. However, breast cancer, which is not uncommon (one in ten women), may disrupt this. and direction may be altered, promoting spread across the midline, into the abdomen, into the vertebrae, up to the cervical nodes or down to the inguinal nodes. Lymph flow may be affected in the axillary nodes causing oedema of the upper limb (lymphoedema).

Respiration

The thorax is for respiration. Its expansion causes lowering of the intrathoracic pressure (creating negative intrapleural pressure), in turn causing air to flow down the only opening into the thorax, the trachea. The diaphragm bulges upward from the abdomen, and its descent increases the vertical diameter of the thorax. Elevation of the ribs increases the anteroposterior (AP) and lateral diameters.

There is dispute over the actions of the intercostal muscles during respiration. It is generally accepted that they prevent indrawing of the chest wall during inspiration and that the external intercostals elevate the ribs for inspiration. The internal intercostal (11) and innermost layers seem to contribute in expiration.

During inspiration the ribs rotate around the axis of their necks (see p. 68). The downward-sloping rib bodies move upward, pushing the sternum upward and forward to increase the AP diameter (pump handle). Those ribs with sloping necks and costal cartilages also splay outward to increase the lateral thoracic diameter. The first four ribs are only able to move upward due to their short, horizontal costal cartilages and, in the case of the first rib, its horizontal neck.

During forced inspiration there is additional eversion of the seventh to tenth ribs, to add a further increase in lateral diameter (bucket handle). This additional movement is carried out by the diaphragm and is only possible in ribs seven to ten, in which the costotransverse facets are flat and permit gliding in addition to the rotation of the neck described above. Any muscle that can aid expansion of the thorax is an accessory muscle of inspiration, for example sternocleidomastoid and pectoralis major. Excessive use of these muscles is most pronounced in disease states, such as asthma.

Expiration, in its quiet phase is passive. It occurs by relaxation and elastic recoil. Forced expiration requires contraction of accessory muscles to compress the thorax, or to compress the abdomen to force the diaphragm upward.

Rib fractures painfully limit respiration. Severe trauma, resulting in fracture of the ribs in more than one place means that the intervening segment 'floats'. It is paradoxically drawn inward on inspiration and forced outward on expiration.

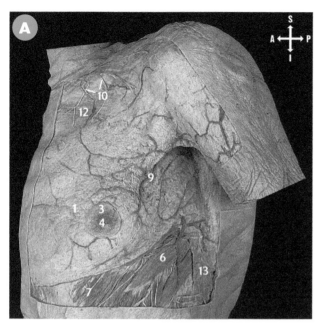

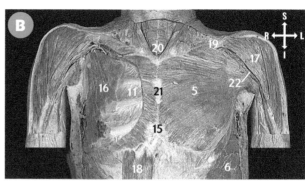

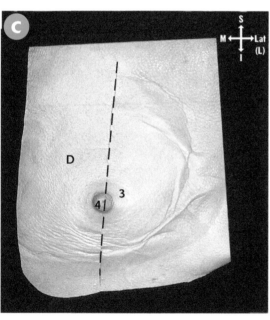

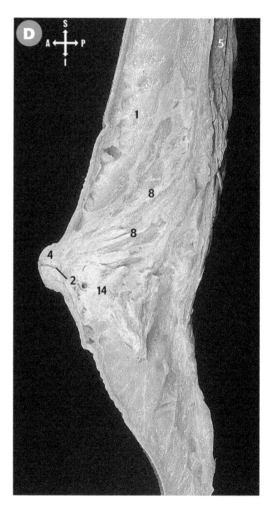

A Superficial dissection of the left breast (from the front and left)
B Muscles of the thoracic wall (from the front)
C Left breast (from the front)
D Sagittal section through the left breast (from the left)

1	Fat of breast	7	External oblique
2	Lactiferous duct	8	Fibrous septae (suspensory
3	Areola of breast		ligaments)
4	Nipple of breast	9	Branches of lateral thoracic artery
5	Pectoralis major	10	Supraclavicular nerves
6	Serratus anterior	11	Internal intercostal muscles

12	Fascia over pectoralis major	18	Rectus abdominis
13	Latissimus dorsi	19	Clavicle
14	Condensed glandular tissue	20	Jugular notch
15	Xiphoid process	21	Body of sternum
16	Pectoralis minor	22	Cephalic vein in deltopectoral
17	Deltoid		groove

Location of numbers: 1AD; 2D; 3AC; 4ACD; 5BD; 6AB; 7A; 8D; 9A; 10A; 11B; 12A; 13A; 14D; 15B; 16B; 17B; 18B; 19B; 20B; 21B; 22B.

Part V

The Abdomen

Full abdomen, peritoneum, position of organs

The abdominal cavity extends upward, inferior to the diaphragm, under the lower ribs and costal margin. It extends inferiorly into the pelvis, and the iliac bones (covered by iliacus and psoas) form the lower aspect of the posterior abdominal wall. The important bony landmarks are: tip of the ninth costal cartilage, particularly the right; anterior superior iliac spine; pubic tubercle; pubic crest; pubic symphysis. The nine regions described during clinical examination of the abdomen are: left and right hypochondrium (**A**); epigastrium (**B**); left and right loin (lumbar) (**C**): umbilical (**D**); left and right iliac fossa (inguinal) (**E**); and suprapubic (**F**).

Peritoneum

Most of the gastro-intestinal tract and associated organs must be able to move and distend. They invaginate a 'balloon' of peritoneum (mesothelium) so that they are covered by visceral peritoneum, but hang on a mesentery (1) arising from the posterior abdominal wall.

The parietal peritoneum extends under the diaphragm, around the abdominal walls and into the pelvis. There is a layer of transversalis fascia between the muscles and the peritoneum. The parietal peritoneum receives sensory supply from the cutaneous nerves of the overlying skin. The phrenic nerves supply the diaphragmatic peritoneum.

The peritoneal cavity is a potential, lubricated space into which blood, fluid and infection may spread rapidly: haemoperitoneum, ascites, peritonitis. Embryonic development of the peritoneal cavity and mesenteries is highly complex. Most organs retain a mesentery posteriorly but some appear to drop out of their mesentery to lie on the posterior abdominal wall retroperitoneally. Those suspended on a mesentery are described as intraperitoneal and any rupture of the viscus will allow its contents to escape into the peritoneal cavity.

During the embryonic stage the lower oesophagus, stomach and first half of the duodenum also have an anterior, ventral mesentery. The liver (2,3) develops in this ventral mesentery, which transmits the umbilical vessels and has a free edge inferiorly. In the adult, the ventral mesentery is the falciform ligament (4), from liver to diaphragm and anterior abdominal wall, and the lesser omentum from liver to stomach (5).

At the epiploic foramen the lesser sac of peritoneum extends behind the stomach and lesser omentum as a diverticulum from the greater sac. It provides a lubricated, potential space for movement and distension of the stomach. It may also be the site of abscess formation or of pancreatic pseudocysts. The epiploic foramen lies behind the free edge of the lesser omentum, in front of the inferior vena cava, above the first part of the duodenum (6) and below the caudate lobe of the liver.

The greater omentum (7) is a fat-filled fold of peritoneum (derived from the embryonic dorsal mesentery of the stomach) that hangs off the inferior edge (greater curvature) of the stomach. It is often called the 'policeman of the abdomen' as it appears to migrate toward, stick to, and seal off diseased organs to prevent their rupture and consequent generalized peritonitis.

Organ positions

The liver and gall bladder (8) lie under the ribs and costal margin above the right hypochondrium. The spleen is high, on the left. The stomach is in the epigastrium. The small intestine lies centrally with much of the duodenum hidden retroperitoneally. The jejunum (9) tends to lie to the upper left and the ileum (10) to the lower right. The ileum may drop into the pelvis.

The first part of the colon, the caecum (11) (with the appendix), is in the right iliac fossa, usually having little or no mesentery. The ascending colon ascends up the right flank, retroperitoneally, in the paravertebral gutter. It turns to become the transverse colon at the hepatic flexure. The transverse colon (12) has its own mesentery that attaches across the abdomen just inferior to the pancreas and duodenum. They both fuse to the undersurface of the greater omentum. In the left hypochondrium, the transverse colon turns as the splenic flexure to become the descending colon that runs in the left flank or paravertebral gutter, behind the peritoneum. It continues as the sigmoid colon, in the left iliac fossa, with a mesentery. The sigmoid colon is mobile on its mesentery, often descending into the pelvis. It becomes the rectum.

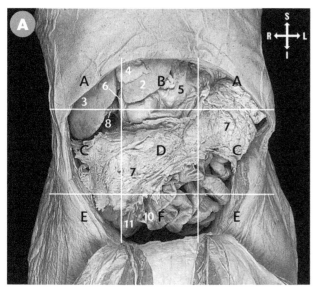

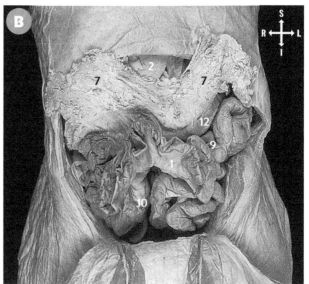

A Abdominal contents (from the front) with grid
   identifying the nine regions of the abdomen
B Abdominal contents with omentum reflected (from the
   front)

The 'nine regions' of the abdomen
A Hypochondrium (left and right)
B Epigastrium
C Lumbar region or loin (left and
   right)
D Umbilical region

E Iliac fossa or inguinal region (left
   and right)
F Hypogastrium or suprapubic
   region

1 Mesentery

2 Left lobe of liver
3 Right lobe of liver
4 Falciform ligament
5 Stomach
6 Superior (first) part of
   duodenum

7 Greater omentum
8 Gall bladder
9 Jejunum
10 Ileum
11 Caecum
12 Transverse colon

Location of numbers: 1B; 2AB; 3A; 4A; 5A; 6A; 7AB; 8A; 9B; 10AB; 11A; 12B.

Lower oesophagus and stomach

Masticated food and fluid pass via the oesophagus to the stomach, a distensible sac that holds and digests food. At its distal end the pyloric sphincter is closed while acid and digestive enzymes are secreted to mix with the food. Muscular action mechanically helps to further mix and digest the food. The pyloric sphincter opens periodically and the resultant chyme is passed into the duodenum.

Lower oesophagus and cardio-oesophageal junction

Having passed through the diaphragm (1), the oesophagus (2) enters the stomach. There is no dissectible, anatomical sphincter at the cardio-oesophageal junction to maintain its closure and prevent reflux of gastric contents into the oesophagus. The right crus of the diaphragm sweeps around the lower end of the oesophagus. There is a resting tone in the circular muscle layer at the lower end of the oesophagus to keep it closed, except during swallowing. The oblique angle at which the oesophagus enters the stomach creates a flap valve, which is elongated and augmented by the extra, oblique layer of muscle in the cardiac region of the stomach wall. All the above contribute to the physiological cardiac sphincter.

A hiatus hernia is where the stomach moves up through the oesophageal diaphragmatic opening (sliding), or a pouch of stomach may pass through the opening to lie alongside the oesophagus (rolling). In the first case, the cardiac sphincter is rendered ineffective. Oesophageal reflux of acidic gastric contents can then occur resulting in pain (heartburn). Erosion of the mucous membrane of the lower oesophagus may follow, which results in oesophagitis.

The oesophageal plexus, formed by the left and right vagus nerves, coalesces into anterior and posterior vagal trunks. These pass through the diaphragm with the oesophagus and continue along the upper lesser curvature (3) of the stomach to supply it, the acid-secreting glands and the pyloric sphincter. Surgically, the oesophagus can be pulled into the abdomen so the vagal trunks may be identified and resected (vagotomy) to control excess acidity or overcome tight closure of the pyloric sphincter.

Portosystemic anastomosis

The gastro-intestinal tract drains to the liver via the portal vein, as does the lower end of the oesophagus (via the left gastric vein). The mid-oesophagus drains to the azygos, part of the systemic circulation. The portal and systemic circulations anastomose via veins in the submucosa of the lower end of the oesophagus. Liver disease may cause portal hypertension, with portal blood escaping via portosystemic anastomoses into the systemic circulation. The submucosal veins involved become dilated to create oesophageal varices, which may rupture and bleed.

Stomach

When empty the stomach is flattened and has a cardia (4), fundus (5), body (6), antrum (7), pylorus (8) and two curvatures, the short upper lesser curvature and the much longer and lower greater curvature (9). The fundus lies posteriorly, to the left of the midline, against the spleen (10) and the diaphragm. On a plain, upright abdominal radiograph a bubble of gas is usually visible in the fundus.

The oesophagus enters obliquely at the cardia. The body curves anteriorly as it passes to the right across the epigastrium. To the right of the midline the body leads to the antrum (the site of greatest acidity) that leads to the pyloric canal, through the pyloric sphincter, close to the tip of the ninth right costal cartilage. The pyloric sphincter is a thickening of the circular muscle layer. It is controlled by vagal (closure) and sympathetic (opening) nerve fibres. Some babies (usually male) are born with hypertrophy of the pyloric sphincter, causing the stomach to overfill and then empty by projectile vomiting (pyloric stenosis).

Arterial supply

An anastomotic ring of blood vessels derived from the coeliac trunk (axis), and its splenic and common hepatic branches, surrounds the stomach. The right and left (12) gastric arteries supply the lesser curvature. The left and right gastro-epiploics supply the greater curvature and the short gastrics supply the fundus and pass from the splenic artery (28) in a double fold of peritoneum that passes from the spleen to the stomach, the gastro-splenic ligament. There are equivalent veins (tributaries of the portal vein). Lymph drainage follows the arteries to the para-aortic nodes around the coeliac trunk.

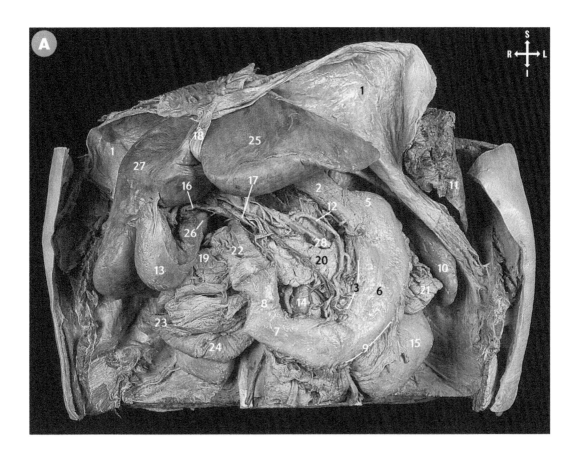

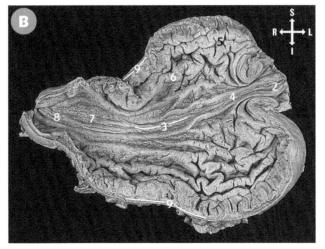

A Upper abdominal contents (from the front)
B Stomach, internal aspect (from the front)

1	Diaphragm	9	Greater curvature of stomach	17	Bile duct
2	Oesophagus	10	Spleen	18	Falciform ligament
3	Lesser curvature of stomach	11	Inferior lobe of left lung	19	Head of pancreas
4	Cardiac region of stomach	12	Left gastric artery	20	Body of pancreas
5	Fundus of stomach	13	Gall bladder	21	Tail of pancreas
6	Body of stomach	14	Aorta	22	Superior (first) part of duodenum
7	Pyloric antrum of stomach	15	Left kidney	23	Descending (second) part of duodenum
8	Pyloric canal of stomach	16	Cystic duct		

24 Horizontal (third) part of duodenum
25 Left lobe of liver
26 Caudate lobe of liver
27 Right lobe of liver
28 Splenic artery

Location of numbers: 1A; 2AB; 3AB; 4B; 5AB; 6AB; 7AB; 8AB; 9AB; 10A; 11A; 12A; 13A; 14A; 15A; 16A; 17A; 18A; 19A; 20A; 21A; 22A; 23A; 24A; 25A; 26A; 27A; 28A.

Intestine

Chyme passes from the stomach (1) into the duodenum (2), where gastric acid is neutralized and further digestive enzymes are added, particularly from the pancreas (3,4,5,6), and bile enters to aid the digestion of fat. Absorption commences in the duodenum, but is the main function of the jejunum and ileum (Illustration B). The mucous membrane of the small intestine is thrown into villi, and the submucosa is thrown into folds (9), all to create a huge, absorptive surface area. The jejunal wall feels thicker than the ileal wall. There are lacteals in the centre of each villus. Digested fats are absorbed via the lacteals and carried in the lymph channels of the mesentery (13) to the cisterna chyli. Other nutrients are absorbed into the blood and carried to the portal vein (14).

The ileum enters the caecum with a valvular effect to prevent reflux from caecum to ileum (ileocaecal valve). The stomach and small intestine secrete large amounts of fluid to mix with the chyme. The colon (large bowel or intestine) is essentially for the reabsorption of that fluid, to dry out what is now waste, and create faeces. Failure to reabsorb the fluid results in diarrhoea. The colonic wall (Illustration D) has no villi and only a few submucosal folds. The epithelium is absorptive, and has many mucus-secreting cells to lubricate the faeces.

The external muscle layer of the large bowel condenses into three strips (taenia coli (17)). The bowel wall tends to bulge between these strips as haustrations or sacculations (18). Tags of fat, appendices epiploicae, hang off the large bowel. These three features help the surgeon differentiate the large from the small bowel. Small pockets or diverticula may develop and extend from the wall of the large bowel, particularly from the sigmoid colon. Such diverticula may become obstructed, inflamed, and even perforate.

Blood supply to most of the intestine is by branches of the superior mesenteric artery (19) until two-thirds of the way around the transverse colon (20). At that point, which is the transition from midgut to hindgut, branches of the inferior mesenteric take over.

Lymphocytes are scattered abundantly throughout the intestinal wall. In the ileum they aggregate as Peyer's patches. The lymphoid tissue has a protective function, and the lymph passes through the mesenteric nodes on its way to the cisterna chyli.

The duodenum has four parts, which form a C-shaped curve around the head of the pancreas. The first part is initially on a short mesentery, but curves to the right and posteriorly (the 'duodenal cap' seen on barium studies) to become retroperitoneal. It lies inferior to the epiploic foramen. The bile duct passes posteromedial to the first part, as does the gastroduodenal artery. Ulcers in the posterior wall of the duodenum may erode into this artery and cause severe bleeding, or erode into the pancreas. Anterior ulcers may perforate into the peritoneal cavity.

The second part of the duodenum (25) is just to the right of the vertebral column (27) and inferior vena cava (28). It overlies the hilum of the right kidney (35). The pancreatic and bile ducts (40) combine to open on its posteromedial wall, as the major duodenal papilla, about two-thirds of the way down. The first part, on its short mesentery is mobile. The second part, retroperitoneal, is fixed. Acceleration and deceleration accidents may cause duodenal rupture at this point. The third part curves over L3, anterior to the inferior vena cava and aorta (41), just inferior to the pancreas and posterior to the superior mesenteric vessels.

The fourth part, just to the left of L2, lifts off the posterior abdominal wall, gains a short mesentery and turns to continue as the jejunum. As it gains a mesentery it may lift folds of peritoneum off the posterior abdominal wall and create peritoneal pockets that may be the sites of internal hernias.

Blood supply

The duodenum is supplied by the superior and inferior pancreaticoduodenal arteries, derived from the coeliac axis and superior mesenteric artery, respectively. Therefore, these latter arteries anastomose in the duodenum. Equivalent veins drain to the portal vein. Lymph drainage follows the arteries to nodes on the aorta around the coeliac axis and superior mesenteric artery.

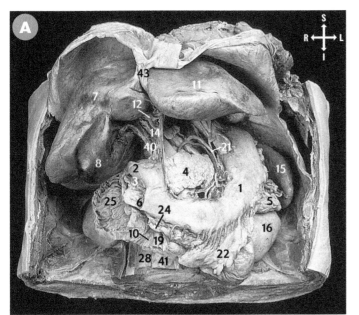

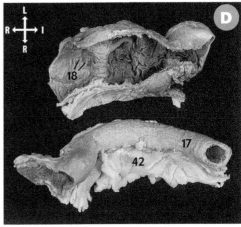

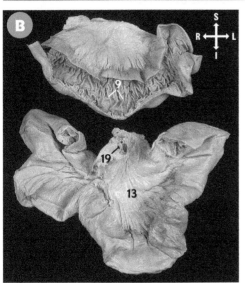

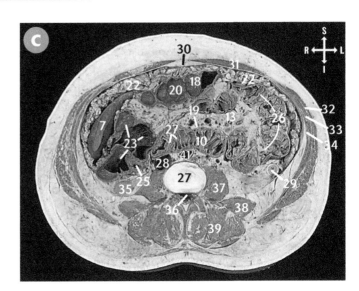

A **Upper abdominal contents (from the front)**
B **Small intestine, external and internal aspect (from the front)**
C **Axial section through the abdomen (from below)**
D **Large intestine, external and internal aspect (from the front)**

1 Body of stomach	11 Left lobe of liver	23 Ascending colon and right colic (hepatic) flexure	32 External oblique
2 Superior (first) part of duodenum	12 Hepatic artery	24 Right gastro-epiploic artery	33 Internal oblique
3 Head of pancreas	13 Mesentery of small bowel	25 Descending (second) part of duodenum	34 Transversus abdominis
4 Body of pancreas	14 Portal vein	26 Jejunum	35 Right kidney lower pole
5 Tail of pancreas	15 Spleen	27 Intervertebral disc between second and third lumbar vertebrae	36 Cauda equina
6 Uncinate process of pancreas	16 Left kidney		37 Psoas major
7 Right lobe of liver	17 Taenia coli	28 Inferior vena cava	38 Quadratus lumborum
8 Gall bladder	18 Haustration/sacculation of colon	29 Descending colon	39 Erector spinae
9 Submucosal folds, plicae circulares	19 Superior mesenteric artery	30 Linea alba	40 Bile duct
10 Horizontal (third) part of duodenum	20 Transverse colon	31 Rectus abdominis	41 Aorta
	21 Left gastric artery		42 Mesentery of sigmoid colon
	22 Greater omentum		43 Falciform ligament

Location of numbers: 1A; 2A; 3A; 4A; 5A; 6A; 7AC; 8A; 9B; 10AC; 11A; 12A; 13BC; 14A; 15A; 16A; 17D; 18CD; 19ABC; 20C; 21A; 22AC; 23C; 24A; 25AC; 26C; 27C; 28AC; 29C; 30C; 31C; 32C; 33C; 34C; 35C; 36C; 37C; 38C; 39C; 40A; 41AC; 42D; 43A.

The (vermiform) appendix, pancreas, spleen

Appendix (vermiform) (Illustration C)

The appendix (1,2) hangs off the caecum (3), below the entry of the ileum (4), at the convergence of the three taenia coli. It is a blind-ended tube of indeterminate function. The appendix is variable in its mesentery (5), its length and its position. It may lie behind or in front of the caecum or the distal end of the ileum, or in the pelvis. The root of the appendix lies at McBurney's point – one-third of the way up a line from the anterior superior iliac spine to the umbilicus.

The lining of the appendix is the same as that of the colon with the addition of nodules of lymphatic tissue. The lumen may become obstructed, and its wall swollen and inflamed. In turn, this inflammation may obstruct the appendicular artery as it runs along the length of the appendix causing gangrene and eventual perforation of the appendix. The variable position may make diagnosis difficult. The early pain of appendicitis usually refers to the midline, in the umbilical region. It then becomes localized in the right iliac fossa as progression of the disease affects the overlying parietal peritoneum. Pus, and/or the contents of a perforated appendix may spread throughout the peritoneal cavity.

Pancreas (Illustration D)

The pancreas secretes digestive enzymes into the duodenum (exocrine). The cells in the islets of Langerhans also have the endocrine function of secreting insulin and glucagon, which control blood sugar. The bile and pancreatic ducts combine to form the hepatopancreatic ampulla (of Vater), which opens in the second part of the duodenum as the major duodenal papilla. There may also be an accessory pancreatic duct that opens at a minor papilla just proximally.

The pancreas is retroperitoneal within the C-shaped curve of the duodenum, and itself curves over the inferior vena cava and aorta before passing toward the hilum of the spleen. It has a head (7), neck (8), body (9) and tail (10). The uncinate process (11) extends from the head and lies posterior to the superior mesenteric vessels. Although most of the pancreas is retroperitoneal, the tail passes into a double fold of peritoneum, which passes between the left kidney and the spleen, the lienorenal ligament.

Blood supply

The splenic artery takes a tortuous course just posterior to the upper edge of the pancreas. It sends many small arteries, as well as the greater pancreatic artery to supply the pancreas, along with the pancreatico-duodenal arteries. The splenic vein is posterior to the pancreas. It meets the superior mesenteric vein to form the portal vein behind the neck of the pancreas.

Pancreatitis is commonly caused by alcohol excess and gallstones. It results in the leakage of pancreatic digestive enzymes into the overlying lesser sac.

Spleen (Illustration A,B)

The spleen has immunological functions. It is a 'blood filter' for old red cells and it stores white blood cells, especially lymphocytes. It lies posteriorly, high in the left upper abdomen, under the diaphragm and above the stomach and left kidney. It is surrounded by peritoneum, and the gastrosplenic and lienorenal ligaments of peritoneum attach it to the stomach and to the posterior abdominal wall, adjacent to the left kidney.

As it lies against the diaphragm the spleen is related to the left ninth, tenth and eleventh ribs. This is extremely significant as fracture of these ribs may rupture the spleen and cause considerable intraperitoneal bleeding. Blood from such a rupture may irritate the left hemidiaphragm and refer pain to the left shoulder tip.

The splenic artery (12) and vein (13) and tail of pancreas reach the hilum of the spleen in the lienorenal ligament. The vessels must be ligated during splenectomy, an operation that may leave the patient susceptible to infection, particularly from *Pneumococcus* and *Haemophilus influenzae*.

The spleen extends anteriorly if it enlarges (congestive cardiac failure, malaria, lymphomas) and it may be palpable at the left costal margin when it is twice its normal size. This superior edge may have a palpable splenic notch (14).

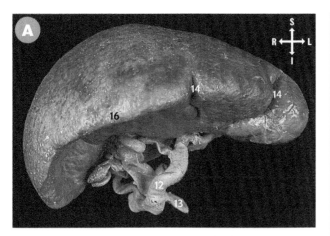

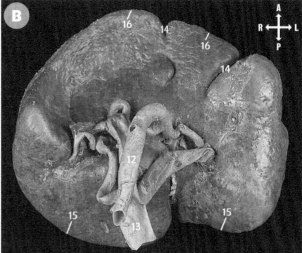

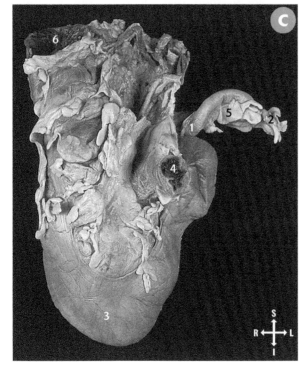

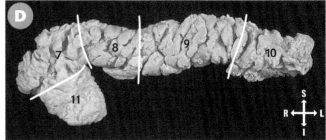

A Spleen (from the front)
B Spleen (from below)

C Caecum and (vermiform) appendix (from the front)
D Pancreas (from the front)

1	Base of (vermiform) appendix	5	Mesentery of appendix	9	Body of pancreas
2	Tip of (vermiform) appendix	6	Ascending colon	10	Tail of pancreas
3	Caecum	7	Head of pancreas	11	Uncinate process of pancreas
4	Terminal ileum	8	Neck of pancreas	12	Splenic artery

13	Splenic vein
14	Notch of spleen
15	Inferior border of spleen
16	Superior border of spleen

Location of numbers: 1C; 2C; 3C; 4C; 5C; 6C; 7D; 8D; 9D; 10D; 11D; 12AB; 13AB; 14AB; 15B; 16AB.

Liver: lobes, surrounding peritoneum and spaces

The liver is the largest gland in the body and has the following functions: produce and secrete bile; metabolise, monitor and maintain blood glucose (glucostat); metabolise and synthesise proteins, amino acids and lipids; store minerals; store and synthesise some vitamins; metabolise and detoxify drugs, toxins and hormones; and – only in the fetus – haemopoiesis.

The liver is a soft, vascular organ that lies high in the abdomen, usually extending across the epigastrium and under the medial edge of the left costal margin. It is a rounded wedge with the base lying posterosuperiorly against the diaphragm and posterior abdominal wall. The 'thin edge' points antero-inferiorly toward the costal margin but should not be palpable below the costal margin in the healthy adult. It is divided into right (1) and left (6) lobes. Anatomically, the right lobe also has caudate (7) (posterior) and quadrate (8) (anterior) lobes. But these are functionally part of the left lobe as they receive blood from the left branches of the portal vein and hepatic artery.

To carry out its functions the liver receives venous blood from the spleen and gastro-intestinal tract via the portal vein. As it is the first organ to receive toxins ingested from the digestive tract it may be particularly susceptible to damage from those toxins. Damage to the liver and/or obstruction to the biliary tree will cause bile pigments to escape from the liver into the blood, causing jaundice, a yellow discoloration of the skin and sclera. Protein synthesis, particularly of plasma proteins and clotting factors, may be disrupted in liver disease, causing such patients to bleed easily. The liver itself is surrounded by a thin fascial capsule, which is not substantial. As a result, it is susceptible to laceration and tearing in deceleration accidents and following fractures of the overlying ribs.

Relations

The gall bladder (9) lies on the undersurface of the liver, between the right and quadrate lobes. The inferior surface of the right lobe is related to the right kidney and suprarenal gland (10), the duodenum (11) and the hepatic flexure of the colon (12). The inferior surface of the left lobe is related to the oesophagus (13) and stomach (14). The quadrate lobe and gall bladder relate to the pylorus and first part of the duodenum.

Peritoneum

In the embryo, the liver forms in the ventral mesentery, but the eventual adult position is as if the liver had invaginated the peritoneum from above and behind. The visceral peritoneum covers the liver and gall bladder and becomes parietal peritoneum as it reflects onto the diaphragm and posterior abdominal wall. The reflections form upper and lower (15) coronary ligaments both on the right and left sides. The left (16) and right (17) triangular ligaments are formed where the respective upper and lower coronary ligaments meet. On the left, the coronary ligaments are so short that the reflections are usually referred to as the left triangular ligament.

The coronary and triangular ligaments surround the bare area of the liver (18) that is related to the inferior vena cava (19), right suprarenal gland and upper pole of the right kidney, lying on the diaphragm as it forms the posterior wall of the upper abdomen.

The falciform ligament (20) separates the liver into its anatomical right and left lobes. The ligamentum teres (21) is the obliterated left umbilical vein, lying in the free edge of the falciform ligament.

Subhepatic and subphrenic potential peritoneal spaces (Illustration A)

The left (A) and right (B) subphrenic spaces are on either side of the falciform ligament, between the liver and the diaphragm. The right subhepatic space (C) is under the right lobe of the liver, between it and the kidney. It communicates with the lesser sac via the epiploic foramen. The left subhepatic space (D) is under the left lobe of the liver, between it and the lesser omentum. The lesser sac, behind the lesser omentum and caudate lobe may also be considered as a subhepatic space.

Theoretically, blood or pus from generalized peritonitis may collect in any of these potential spaces. The right subhepatic space is the most common (as patients are usually recumbent) with the possible consequence of abscess formation.

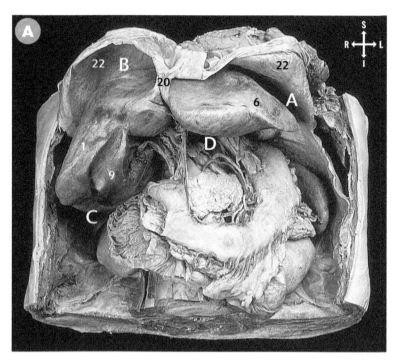

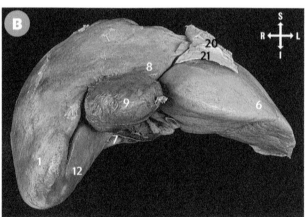

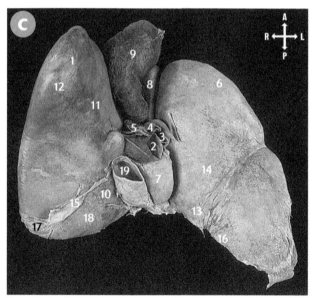

A Upper abdominal contents (from the front)
B Liver (from the front)
C Liver (from below)

Abdominal spaces	1	Right lobe of liver	10	Position of right kidney and suprarenal gland in relation to the undersurface of the liver
A Left subphrenic space	2	Portal vein		
B Right subphrenic space	3	Hepatic artery		
C Right subhepatic or hepatorenal space (pouch of Rutherford Morison)	4	Common hepatic duct	11	Position of duodenum in relation to the undersurface of the liver
	5	Cystic duct		
	6	Left lobe of liver	12	Position of colon in relation to the undersurface of the liver
D Left subhepatic space	7	Caudate lobe of liver		
	8	Quadrate lobe of liver	13	Position of oesophagus in relation to the undersurface of the liver
	9	Gall bladder		

14	Position of stomach in relation to the undersurface of the liver
15	Lower right coronary ligament
16	Left triangular ligament
17	Right triangular ligament
18	Bare area of liver
19	Inferior vena cava
20	Falciform ligament
21	Position of ligamentum teres
22	Diaphragm

Location of numbers: 1ABC; 2C; 3C; 4C; 5C; 6ABC; 7BC; 8BC; 9ABC; 10C; 11C; 12BC; 13C; 14C; 15C; 16C; 17C; 18C; 19C; 20AB; 21B; 22A.

Gall bladder, biliary tree, porta hepatis

Biliary system

Bile is formed continually in the liver. It is stored and concentrated in the gall bladder that then releases bile when necessary in response to a fatty meal, usually mediated by the release of cholecystokinin.

The gall bladder (2), covered by peritoneum, lies in a fossa (bare of peritoneum) between the right (3) and quadrate (4) lobes of the liver. It has a fundus (5), body (6) and neck (7). The cystic duct (8) passes from the neck of the gall bladder to join the common hepatic duct (9). As the two ducts join, they continue as the bile duct. The mucous membrane at the gall bladder neck folds and overlaps to form the spiral valve. The cystic artery (12), which is usually a branch of the right hepatic, supplies the gall bladder, but variations are common. Venous drainage is to the portal vein. Arterial anomalies are not uncommon in this area, e.g. the common hepatic artery, usually from the coeliac, may occasionally arise from the superior mesenteric.

The bile duct lies in front of the portal vein and to the right of the hepatic artery in the free edge of the lesser omentum. Just behind and to the left of the first part of the duodenum it is related to the gastroduodenal artery. But the duct then runs through the head of the pancreas, to join the pancreatic duct and enter the second part of the duodenum at the major duodenal papilla. The sphincter of Oddi has three parts, one around the lower bile duct, one around the pancreatic duct (to prevent bile entering the pancreas), and one around the combined duct just before the ampulla. If bile is not required the sphincter closes and bile cannot escape down the bile duct. Instead is passes via the cystic duct to the gall bladder. When the sphincter is open flow reverses down the cystic duct and into the bile duct, to the duodenum.

 The gall bladder is susceptible to stone formation and consequent inflammation – cholecystitis. Pain may refer to the epigastrium, in the midline. However, if the inflamma-tion reaches the peritoneum on the undersurface of the diaphragm, it is detected by the phrenic nerve (C3,4,5) and may refer to the right shoulder tip. Pain may be elicited directly from an inflamed gall bladder by asking a patient to inhale while palpating beneath the costal margin at the tip of the ninth right costal cartilage. Pain is a positive Murphy's sign.

Jaundice has a number of causes. Pre-hepatic jaundice is an overload of bilirubin (despite a normal liver) usually because of excessive blood breakdown (haemolytic jaundice). Hepatic jaundice is a result of damage to the liver's cellular structure (hepatitis, cirrhosis). Post-hepatic jaundice is due to obstruction of the hepatic and/or bile ducts causing biliary back pressure into the liver and the leakage of conjugated bilirubin into the blood.

Gallstones that migrate from the gall bladder and into the bile duct may cause painful, intermittent jaundice. Carcinoma of the head of the pancreas, obstructing the bile duct from its outside, may cause painless, continuous jaundice. A stone obstructing the major duodenal papilla may cause bile to flow back into the pancreas via the pancreatic duct to cause pancreatitis.

Porta hepatis and neurovascular supply

At the porta hepatis the portal vein (13) and hepatic artery (14) divide into left and right branches to enter the liver. The left (15) and right (16) hepatic ducts carry bile from the liver and converge to form the (common) hepatic duct. The artery also brings autonomic innervation and has parallel lymph drainage, which eventually returns to nodes around the coeliac trunk. Lymph nodes at the porta may enlarge and obstruct biliary flow.

Blood from the portal vein (full of nutrients but deoxygenated) and the hepatic artery (oxygenated) filter through the liver to converge on a variable number (two to four) of hepatic veins that drain directly into the inferior vena cava. The (hepatic) portal vein is formed by the splenic and superior mesenteric veins. The inferior mesenteric usually joins the splenic, but may join the superior mesenteric or join the portal vein just as it is formed.

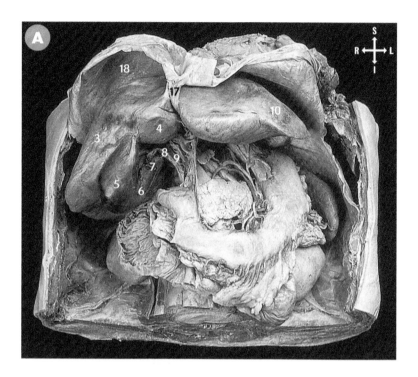

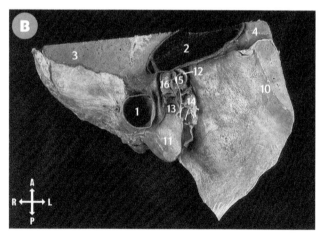

A Upper abdominal contents (from the front)
B Liver, with gall bladder in coronal section (from below)

1	Inferior vena cava	**6**	Body of gall bladder	**11**	Caudate lobe of liver	**16**	Right hepatic duct
2	Gall bladder	**7**	Neck of gall bladder	**12**	Cystic artery	**17**	Falciform ligament
3	Right lobe of liver	**8**	Cystic duct	**13**	Portal vein	**18**	Diaphragm
4	Quadrate lobe of liver	**9**	Common hepatic duct	**14**	Hepatic artery		
5	Fundus of gall bladder	**10**	Left lobe of liver	**15**	Left hepatic duct		

Location of numbers: 1B; 2B; 3AB; 4AB; 5A; 6A; 7A; 8A; 9A; 10AB; 11B; 12B; 13B; 14B; 15B; 16B; 17A; 18A.

Kidneys

The kidneys lie retroperitoneally, high on the posterior abdominal wall. They filter the blood to produce urine. They are vital to the control of plasma sodium level and of blood pressure via the secretion of renin. Renal disease often leads to hypertension. The kidneys also synthesize erythropoietin, which stimulates the bone marrow to produce red blood cells and hydroxycholecalciferol (a derivative of vitamin D), which is important for maintaining serum calcium levels.

Renal fat (Illustration A) is the term often used to include the perirenal fat, renal fascia and pararenal fat. A thin, tough capsule (2) immediately surrounds the kidney, which is a delicate organ and therefore surrounded, and protected, by further layers of fat and fascia.

Perirenal fat is immediately outside the kidney capsule. Renal fascia encloses the kidney, suprarenal (adrenal) gland (3) and perirenal fat (4). It is derived from, and is continuous with the transversalis fascia. The renal fascia is closely applied to the upper and lateral aspects of the kidney. But perirenal effusions may extend into its potential space inferiorly and medially. Pararenal fat surrounds the kidney and adrenal, outside the renal fascia. It usually has a firmer consistency than fat elsewhere in the body.

Relations

The hilum of the left kidney is at L1, and the right at L2. They cause an indentation or sinus on the medial border of the kidney (Illustration B). The right kidney is slightly lower than the left, being displaced by the liver. From its hilum, which is anteromedial, the kidney falls backward and laterally into the paravertebral gutter alongside psoas major. The upper aspects of the kidneys are related to the eleventh and twelfth ribs, and therefore lie on the diaphragm, moving on respiration. When attempting to palpate an enlarged kidney it is necessary to ask the patient to inhale. When operating

on the kidney care must be taken not to incise the diaphragm and possibly create a pneumothorax. Occasionally the diaphragm may be deficient posteriorly. The kidney is then directly related to the pleura.

As the kidney is retroperitoneal most of its anterior relations are separated from it by the peritoneum. But structures that are also retroperitoneal are directly related the kidney and its renal fat. On the right the liver is anterior to the kidney, with the peritoneal pouch of Rutherford Morison between. The upper pole of the kidney is directly related to the bare area of the liver. Medially the duodenum (second part) is directly related to the kidney and its hilum, whereas the ascending colon is similarly related to the lower pole.

On the left the tail of the pancreas and the splenic vessels (5) directly cross the hilum of the kidney. The descending colon (6) is directly related to the lower lateral pole. The stomach (7), spleen (8) and jejunum (9) are anterior relations, but with peritoneum in between. The lesser sac extends between the stomach and left kidney.

Internally, the kidney shows a peripheral cortex (10) around a medulla (11). The latter has pyramids (12), which become renal papillae that push into minor calyces (13), the first part of the urinary collecting/conducting system. The minor calyces converge into two or three major calyces (14), which themselves converge to form the renal pelvis (15).

Neurovascular supply

The hilum of the kidney has the renal vein (16) (or its branches) anteriorly, the renal pelvis becoming ureter (17) posteriorly, and the renal artery (18), with its variable branches in the middle. The inferior vena cava (IVC) is to the right of the midline, therefore the right renal vein is much shorter than the left. When operating on the right kidney it is possible to tear the short renal vein from the IVC.

Nerves are derived from the coeliac plexus. Lymph drains to para-aortic nodes.

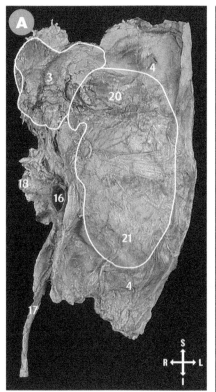

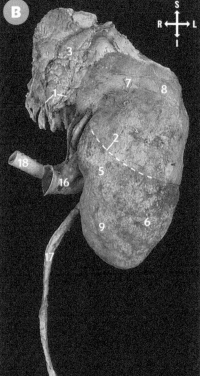

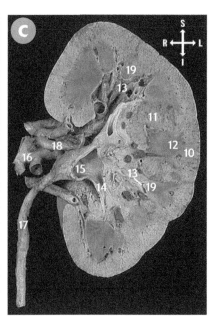

A Left kidney, encapsulated in fat (from the front)
B The left kidney from the front
C The left kidney in coronal section from the front

1 Suprarenal vessels	**6** Position of descending colon in	**9** Position of jejunum in relation to	**15** Renal pelvis
2 Cut border of fibrous capsule	relation to the anterior surface of	the anterior surface of the	**16** Renal vein
(inferior portion removed)	the kidney	kidney	**17** Ureter
3 Suprarenal (adrenal) gland	**7** Position of stomach in relation to	**10** Renal cortex	**18** Renal artery
4 Perinephric (perirenal) fat	the anterior surface of the kidney	**11** Renal medulla	**19** Renal papilla
5 Position of tail of pancreas and	**8** Position of spleen in relation to	**12** Medullary pyramid	**20** Position of upper pole of kidney
splenic vessels in relation to the	the anterior surface of the	**13** Minor calyx	**21** Position of lower pole of kidney
anterior surface of the kidney	kidney	**14** Major calyx	

Location of numbers: **1**B; **2**B; **3**AB; **4**A; **5**B; **6**B; **7**B; **8**B; **9**B; **10**C; **11**C; **12**C; **13**C; **14**C; **15**C; **16**ABC; **17**ABC; **18**ABC; **19**C; **20**A; **21**A.

Ureter, suprarenal (adrenal) gland

Ureter

The ureter leaves the renal pelvis to run retroperitoneally down the posterior abdominal wall. It is a muscular tube lined by urinary transitional epithelium and peristaltic waves propel the urine to the bladder. If touched during surgery, the ureter will contract and appear to 'worm' on the posterior abdominal wall.

The ureter (1) lies on psoas major (3), posterior to all other structures except the genitofemoral nerve (4). It crosses the bifurcation of the common iliac artery (5) to enter the pelvis, then down and forward to the bladder, which it enters obliquely to prevent reflux. The right ureter passes behind the second part of the duodenum (6), the right colic and iliac vessels, the gonadal vessels, and the root of the mesentery. The left ureter also lies behind the gonadal vessels, as well as the left colic vessels and the root of the sigmoid mesentery. The ureter is visualized on a plain abdominal radiograph as lateral to the tips of the lumbar transverse processes, anterior to the sacro-iliac joint and medial to the ischial spine.

The ureter is supplied by the vessels that are adjacent to it, and they also carry its nerve supply: renal, gonadal, iliac, and vesical or uterine.

Ureteric stones are not uncommon and may pass down the ureter, referring severe pain to the loin and groin as well as to the tip of the penis in the male. There are supposedly three narrowings where stones may be delayed, the pelvi-ureteric junction, the pelvic brim, and the passage of the ureter through the bladder wall, but these narrowings are debatable.

Suprarenal (adrenal) glands (Illustration B)

The suprarenal glands lie at the upper, medial pole of each kidney, within the renal fascia. They are endocrine glands with a peripheral cortex and an internal medulla.

The suprarenal medulla is like a modified sympathetic ganglion in that under the stimulation of preganglionic sympathetic nerves it secretes adrenaline and noradrenaline. The resultant sudden rise of these hormones, usually in response to danger or stress gives the typical 'fight or flight' response: increased cardiac rate and output; widely staring eyes with dilated pupils; an inhibition of gastro-intestinal activity; and many other sympathetic responses associated with a sudden fright.

The suprarenal cortex is essential to life and involved in the body's reaction to stress. It has three layers that secrete different hormones. Aldosterone acts on the kidney for the maintenance of sodium and potassium levels. Cortisol and corticosterone affect carbohydrate metabolism, the body's connective tissues and the immune system. Sex hormones, particularly the male androgens, are secreted, but normally in insignificant amounts.

Both glands lie retroperitoneally on the crura of the diaphragm. The lesser sac and stomach are anterior to the left suprarenal, while the bare area of the liver and inferior vena cava (IVC) are related to the right.

Each gland is supplied by branches from three arteries, but drained by one large vein. On the right the vein is short and enters the IVC, whereas on the left, the suprarenal vein enters the left renal vein. The suprarenals receive an abundant nerve supply from the splanchnic nerves and coeliac plexus, which lies between them.

Tumours may be found in both the cortex and medulla. If the medulla is affected the symptoms are those of massive stimulation of the sympathetic system (phaeochromocytoma). Should the glands fail, or require surgical removal the patient must regularly take corticosteroid drugs.

The IVC (7) is to the right of the midline, therefore, the right suprarenal and right gonadal veins drain into it. The left suprarenal and gonadal veins (8) drain into the left renal vein (9), which passes anterior to the aorta, but behind the superior mesenteric artery, behind the pancreas, above the third part of the duodenum. The IVC lies to the right of the aorta, the left common iliac vein passes behind the right common iliac artery.

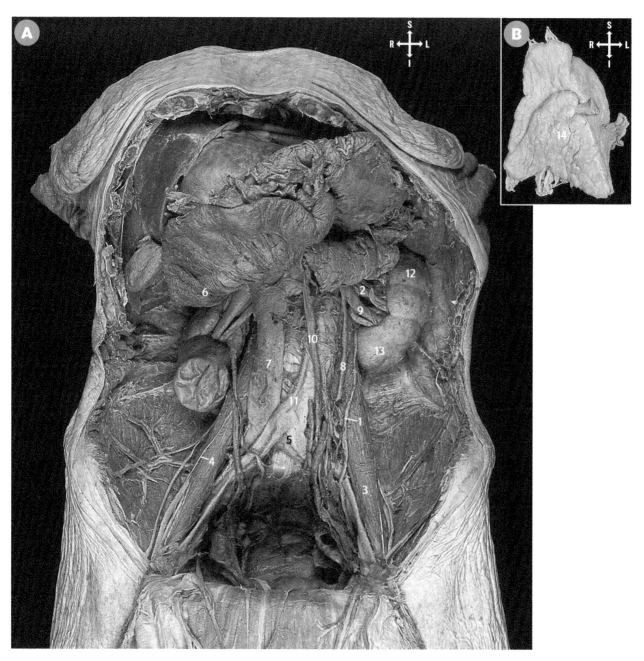

A   Posterior abdominal wall (from the front)
B   Left suprarenal gland (from the front)

1	Ureter	5	Common iliac artery and vein	8	Gonadal vein	12	Upper pole of kidney

1   Ureter
2   Renal artery
3   Psoas major
4   Genitofemoral nerve

5   Common iliac artery and vein
6   Descending (second part) of
    duodenum reflected superiorly
7   Inferior vena cava

8   Gonadal vein
9   Renal vein
10 Inferior mesenteric vein
11 Aorta

12 Upper pole of kidney
13 Lower pole of kidney
14 Left suprarenal (adrenal) gland

Location of numbers: 1A; 2A; 3A; 4A; 5A; 6A; 7A; 8A; 9A; 10A; 11A; 12A; 13A; 14B.

Posterior abdominal wall muscles, mesentery

The posterior abdominal wall includes the diaphragm, psoas major and iliacus, quadratus lumborum and transversus abdominis. The individual muscles are surrounded by their fascial sheaths (epimysium) and they are all overlain internally by variable, often indistinguishable, transversalis fascia.

The vertebral column (T12–L5) is prominent in the midline, with the aorta and inferior vena cava on its anterior surface. On either side are two paravertebral gutters. The convexity of the lumbar vertebrae pushes into the abdomen, therefore, structures passing transversely across the posterior abdominal wall must curve over the vertebrae.

Muscles and nerves

Psoas major (1) lies on each side of the vertebral column, arising from the five lumbar vertebrae, their intervening discs and the transverse processes. It passes inferiorly to join iliacus (2), arising from the internal aspect of the iliac bone, and form the iliopsoas tendon that inserts onto the lesser trochanter of the femur. Iliopsoas is a hip flexor. Psoas is supplied segmentally by L1–4 and iliacus by the femoral nerve.

The lumbar plexus is formed within psoas by the ventral rami of T12–L5. The resultant nerves emerge onto the posterior abdominal (and pelvic) walls in an extremely variable pattern but usually described as: subcostal T12; ilio-inguinal (3) and iliohypogastric L1; lateral cutaneous nerve of thigh (lateral femoral cutaneous) (4) L2,3; genitofemoral L1,2; femoral L2,3,4; obturator L2,3,4; and lumbosacral trunk L4,5. The subcostal, ilio-inguinal and iliohypogastric nerves supply the lower parts of the abdominal wall muscles, and the skin of the lower abdomen and anterior aspect of the genitalia. The others pass to the skin and muscles of the thigh and leg.

Quadratus lumborum (5) attaches to the posterior iliac crest, the twelfth rib and the lumbar transverse processes. It stabilizes and laterally flexes the vertebral column. It fixes the twelfth rib during deep inspira-

tion. With its neighbour, quadratus lumborum extends the vertebral column. The nerve supply is segmental, T12–L3.

Transversus abdominis (6) arises from: the internal aspect of the lower six costal cartilages; the thoracolumbar fascia (which is a strong fascia around erector spinae and quadratus lumborum); the iliac crest; and the inguinal ligament. It runs horizontally around the abdomen to insert into the rectus sheath and linea alba. It acts with the other abdominal wall muscles to support and compress the abdominal viscera. The nerve supply is segmental, T7–L1.

Mesentery

The mesentery (7) is a fan-shaped double fold of peritoneum that contains a variable amount of fat along with the superior mesenteric artery, vein and associated nerves, lymph vessels and lymph nodes.

The root (origin) of the mesentery is 15 cm long. It starts to the left of L2 and passes obliquely downward and to the right, to end opposite the right sacro-iliac joint. It crosses: the fourth and third parts of the duodenum; the aorta, where the superior mesenteric artery enters it; the inferior vena cava; and the right ureter. The distal end is approximately 6 m long to accommodate the length of the jejunum and ileum.

Within the mesentery the superior mesenteric artery splays into jejunal, ileal and caecal branches. It has already sent the middle colic artery into the mesentery of the transverse colon, and will send the right colic artery, retroperitoneally to the ascending colon. The jejunal and ileal branches anastomose with each other in a series of arterial arcades. The jejunum has few arcades, with long vessels passing to it. The ileum has multiple arcades, with short vessels passing to it. This pattern, along with the fact that the jejunal mesentery has less fat than the ileal, may help the surgeon identify the parts of the bowel. Equivalent veins converge on the superior mesenteric vein.

The lymph nodes within the mesentery may become infected and enlarged. The blood vessels may become occluded and in spite of the anastomotic arcades, part of the bowel may become ischaemic.

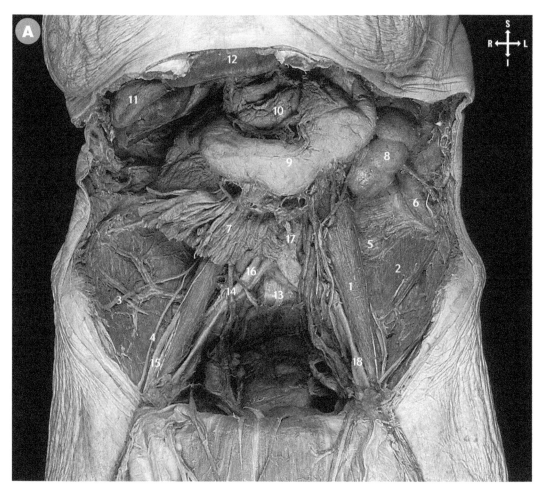

A Posterior abdominal wall (from the front)

1	Psoas major	6	Transversus abdominis	11	Gall bladder	
2	Iliacus	7	Mesentery	12	Left lobe of liver	
3	Ilio-inguinal nerve	8	Kidney	13	Promontory of sacrum	
4	Lateral cutaneous nerve of thigh	9	Stomach	14	Ureter	
5	Quadratus lumborum	10	Body of pancreas	15	Femoral nerve	

16 Common iliac artery and vein
17 Aorta
18 External iliac artery and vein

Anterior abdominal wall

On each side, the anterior abdominal wall has one longitudinal muscle, rectus abdominis (1), and three that sweep around it, become aponeurotic and contribute to the rectus sheath (2) before fusing in the linea alba (3). They pass from the thoracic cage to the pelvis, and have the following functions: abdominal compression to raise the intra-abdominal pressure during defecation, micturition, parturition and forced expiration, including coughing and sneezing; support of the abdominal contents; and support, flexion and lateral flexion of the lumbar vertebral column.

External to the muscular layers the superficial fascia has a distinct membranous layer that thickens inferiorly as Scarpa's fascia to support the weight of the viscera. Internally, a layer of transversalis fascia lies between the musculature and the parietal peritoneum.

Surgical incisions are frequently made through the abdominal wall. It is important to know the directions of the muscle fibres, and the positions and directions of the neurovascular bundles to understand why some incisions are used. Inferiorly, the inguinal canal is a potential site of hernias (see pp. 168 and 169).

External oblique (4) (T7–12) arises from the lower eight ribs (interdigitating with serratus anterior and latissimus dorsi). It passes inferomedially, with a free posterior margin, to the outer lip of the anterior half of the iliac crest. At the anterior superior iliac spine (ASIS) (5) it forms an aponeurosis that in rolls between the ASIS and the pubic tubercle (6) as the inguinal ligament (7). At the pubic tubercle, the inguinal ligament curves back upon itself as the lacunar ligament, to reach the pectineal line and end as the pectineal ligament. The superficial inguinal ring (8) is an opening in the aponeurosis, immediately above the pubic crest. The muscle fibres become aponeurotic at a line between the ASIS and the umbilicus (9). One-third of the way up this line is 'McBurney's point'

(10), the site of incision for appendicectomy.

Internal oblique (11) (T7–L1) is deep to external oblique and the muscle fibres are at right angles to it,

running superomedially. Internal oblique attaches to the costal margin, the lumbar fascia, the iliac crest and the lateral two-thirds of the inguinal ligament. The fibres arising from the ligament arch over the inguinal canal and fuse with similarly arching fibres of transversus abdominis to form the conjoint tendon.

Transversus abdominis (12) (T7–L1) forms the deepest muscle layer. The fibres run transversely and attach to the lower six ribs and costal cartilages (interdigitating with the diaphragm), the lumbar fascia, the iliac crest and the lateral half or one-third of the inguinal ligament. These lower fibres arch over the inguinal canal to form the conjoint tendon. The conjoint tendon is continuous with the anterior rectus sheath and attaches to the pubic crest and medial end of the pectineal line, behind the superficial inguinal ring.

The inferior epigastric artery, with accompanying veins (13) arises from the external iliac at the mid-inguinal point, which is just medial to the mid point of the inguinal ligament. It ascends towards the umbilicus and enters the rectus sheath (14) where it anastomoses with the superior epigastric artery. The inferior epigastric is at risk during the insertion of instruments for laparoscopy.

The neurovascular bundles in the seventh to eleventh intercostal spaces, the subcostal bundle inferior to the twelfth rib, and branches of the L1 spinal nerve, curve inferomedially around the abdominal wall between internal oblique and transversus abdominis. They send cutaneous branches, segmentally, to the skin, parietal peritoneum, and the muscles. At a variable distance anterior to the ASIS they pierce internal oblique to run posterior to the aponeurosis of external oblique. The ilio-inguinal branch of L1 is at a lower level, just above the inguinal ligament. As it passes to lie deep to external oblique it is in the inguinal canal and emerges from the superficial ring to supply adjacent skin.

Surgical incisions should avoid cutting the nerves, and any reflection of rectus abdominis should be done in a lateral direction – towards the nerves that are entering and supplying it (see pp. 167 and 169).

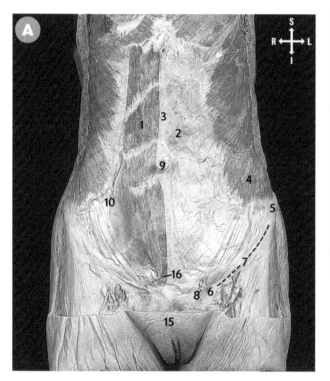

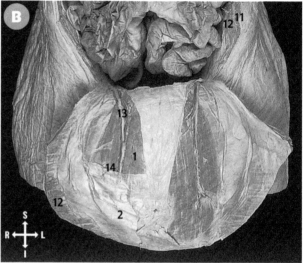

A Muscles of the anterior abdominal wall, external (from the front)

B Muscles of the anterior abdominal wall, internal (from below)

1	Rectus abdominis	6	Pubic tubercle	11	Internal oblique	15	Mons pubis
2	Rectus sheath	7	Position of inguinal ligament	12	Transversus abdominis	16	Pyramidalis
3	Linea alba	8	Superficial inguinal ring	13	Inferior epigastric artery and vein		
4	External oblique	9	Umbilicus	14	Arcuate line, free edge of		
5	Anterior superior iliac spine	10	McBurney's point		posterior rectus sheath		

Location of numbers: 1AB; 2AB; 3A; 4A; 5A; 6A; 7A; 8A; 9A; 10A; 11B; 12B; 13B; 14B; 15A; 16A.

Part VI

The Male and Female Pelvis

Pelvic floor, ischio-anal fossa

The pelvic cavity is superior to the muscular pelvic floor (or diaphragm), and the perineum is inferior to it. The sacrospinous ligament (1) gives origin to some of the pelvic floor muscles. The lesser sciatic foramen (2) lies inferior to the ligament, therefore inferior to the pelvic floor. Nerves and vessels passing through the lesser sciatic foramen enter the perineum, as do structures that pass through the pelvic floor.

Pelvic floor muscles

The lateral wall of the true pelvis gives origin to obturator internus (3), a lateral rotator of the hip. The muscle is covered by obturator fascia that has a thickened 'white line' (4) running from the ischial spine to the pubic body. The pelvic floor supports the pelvic organs. The floor must not only expand, but also contract, as it contributes to the sphincteric control of some of the emerging organs, and therefore, it must be muscular.

Coccygeus and levator ani arise in continuity with each other; coccygeus (5) from the sacrum, coccyx and sacrospinous ligament; levator ani (6) from the ischial spine, white line of obturator fascia and posterior aspect of the body of the pubis. Both muscles pass downward and medially to form a midline raphe that passes from the coccyx (7) to the pubic symphysis (8). The raphe is thickened between the coccyx and anal canal as the anococcygeal ligament (9) and anterior to the anal canal as the perineal body, or central tendon of the perineum. The raphe is pierced by the anal canal (10), urethra (11) and, in the female, the vagina.

Levator ani is subdivided into iliac and pubic parts. Iliococcygeus and pubococcygeus insert into the coccyx and anococcygeal ligament. Puborectalis loops around the anorectal junction to fuse with its neighbour from the other side and draw the anorectal junction up and forward. Pubovaginalis loops around the vagina to create a sphincteric effect around both it and the urethra. In the male pubovaginalis is replaced by levator prostatae that supports the prostate gland.

The perineal branches of S3 and S4 supply levator ani, along with branches from the pudendal nerve (S2,3,4). Branches of S5 supply coccygeus.

During childbirth the pelvic floor and/or perineal body may be damaged. Tears may need to be sutured, and pelvic floor exercises become necessary to rebuild supportive muscle tone. Laxity of the pelvic floor may allow the pelvic organs to slip from their normal anatomical positions, possibly compromising urinary control, leading to incontinence. In extreme cases the pelvic organs may prolapse into and even right out of the vagina.

Perineum

The diamond-shaped perineum is bounded by: the ischial tuberosities (12), covered by obturator internus and obturator fascia; the sacrotuberous ligaments (13); the ischiopubic rami (14); and the inferior end of the pubic symphysis. It is divided into a posterior anal triangle and an anterior urogenital triangle. The ischio-anal fossa (15) is a pyramid with its base covered by skin, its lateral aspect formed by obturator fascia, and its medial aspect formed by levator ani and the anal canal surrounded by its external sphincter. It is filled with fat to allow distension of the anal canal during defecation.

The pudendal neurovascular bundle (16) of internal pudendal artery and vein, and the pudendal nerve (S2,3,4), leaves the pelvis to enter the buttock by passing between piriformis (17) and coccygeus. It then curves around the ischial spine and sacrospinous ligament to enter the ischio-anal fossa, lying on its lateral wall in a fascial (Alcock's) canal on obturator internus. It passes forward to supply the perineal structures. The inferior rectal neurovascular bundle (18) arises high up in the fossa and runs on levator ani to supply the anal sphincter and sensation to the anal canal.

The fat in the fossa is prone to infection and abscess formation. Such an abscess may extend forward into a recess between the pelvic floor and the deep perineal pouch, the anterior recess of the ischio-anal fossa.

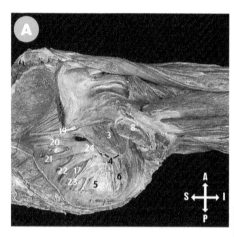

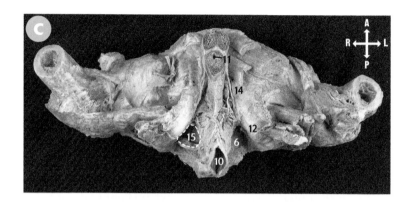

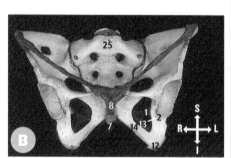

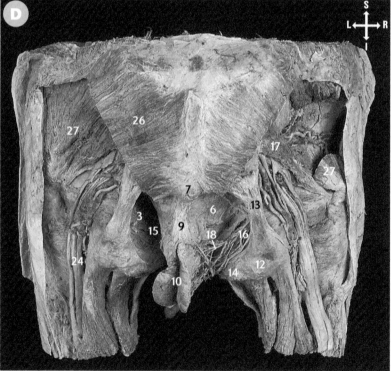

A Left pelvic floor (from the right)
B Bones and ligaments of the pelvis (from the front)
C Male perineum (from below)
D Female ischio-anal region (from behind)

1	Sacrospinous ligament	8	Pubic symphysis
2	Lesser sciatic foramen	9	Anococcygeal ligament
3	Obturator internus	10	Anal canal
4	Obturator fascia, white line, origin of levator ani	11	Urethra
5	Coccygeus	12	Ischial tuberosity
6	Levator ani	13	Sacrotuberous ligament
7	Coccyx	14	Ischiopubic ramus
		15	Ischio-anal fossa

16	Pudendal artery, vein and nerve
17	Piriformis
18	Inferior rectal artery, vein and nerve
19	Obturator nerve
20	Lumbosacral trunk
21	Ventral ramus of first sacral nerve

22	Ventral ramus of second sacral nerve
23	Ventral ramus of third sacral nerve
24	Left sciatic nerve
25	Promontory of sacrum
26	Gluteus maximus
27	Gluteus medius

Location of numbers: 1B; 2B; 3AD; 4A; 5A; 6ACD; 7BD; 8AB; 9D; 10CD; 11C; 12BCD; 13BD; 14BCD; 15CD; 16D; 17AD; 18D; 19A; 20A; 21A; 22A; 23A; 24AD; 25B; 26D; 27D.

Urogenital triangle, external genitalia

The urogenital triangle has deep and superficial perineal pouches, above and below the perineal membrane, a triangular sheet of fascia (stronger in the male to support the penis) that attaches to the ischiopubic rami to span the sub-pubic angle. In the midline the base of the membrane attaches to the perineal body (1).

The deep perineal pouch or urogenital diaphragm is a 'sandwich' of fascia and muscle. The perineal membrane is the outer, inferior layer. The external urethral sphincter and the deep transverse perineal muscles that help fix and stabilize the structures within the region, lie above it. The fascia on the superior surface of these muscles forms the deeper, superior layer of the pouch. The superficial perineal pouch is inferior or superficial to the perineal membrane and contains the external genitalia.

The scrotum houses both testes, so that they lie outside the body cavity, at a slightly lower temperature. The skin is rugose (2), darker than skin elsewhere and is covered with pubic hair. There is a midline raphe, which stops at the anus (3), but continues with the raphe on the ventral surface of the penis. The superficial fascia (Colles') is fat free, continuous with the similar layer in the penis, abdominal wall and upper thigh, but it fuses with the perineal body. It contains dartos muscle (4) that contracts during cold or exercise to raise the testes closer to the body (see p. 168).

The labia majus (5) are thick folds of skin that meet anteriorly over the pubic symphysis as the mons pubis (6). Posteriorly they narrow and meet in the posterior commissure (7). Externally the mons and labia are covered by pubic hair. Internally the skin becomes thinner and is pink and moist. The thickness of each labium is created by fibro-fatty tissue, into which the round ligament of the uterus inserts.

Vascular supply is via the external pudendal arteries and veins anteriorly, and the posterior scrotal or labial branches of the internal pudendal arteries and veins posteriorly. Lymph drainage is to the superficial inguinal nodes.

Scrotal and labial nerve supply is also divided into the anterior third and posterior two-thirds. In the scrotum these sensory nerves carry sympathetic fibres to dartos. The ilio-inguinal and genital branch of genitofemoral are anterior (L1). The posterior scrotal or labial branches of the pudendal (S2,3,4) and the perineal branches of the femoral cutaneous nerve of the thigh (S2,3) are posterior.

The labia minora are thin, fat-free folds of pink, moist skin that lie within, and hidden by the labia majora. Posteriorly they fade by merging with the labia majora. Anteriorly they split into lateral and medial folds, which fuse with those from the opposite side to form the prepuce of the clitoris (8).

The vaginal vestibule, between the labia minora, is covered by similar pink, moist skin. The vaginal opening (9) is small in the young and incompletely closed by the hymen. Occasionally the hymen completely closes the vagina. Such closure may only become apparent at puberty with the commencement of menstruation. Once the hymen has been ruptured it is visible only as a few folds of skin, the carunculae hymenales, at the vaginal opening. The slit-like urethral opening (10) is immediately anterior to the vaginal opening.

The bulbs of the vestibule (11) are the equivalent of the penile bulb (p. 112), but are divided into two halves by the vagina and urethra. Each bulb of erectile tissue is overlain by bulbospongiosus muscle. They are attached to the superficial surface of the perineal membrane, meeting only in an anterior commissure in front of the urethra. Their function is uncertain. Hidden under the posterior end of each bulb is a greater vestibular (Bartholin) gland (13) that opens into the vaginal opening or the immediately adjacent vestibule. These secrete lubricating mucus and are aided by para-urethral and lesser vestibular glands, whose secretions reach the vestibule via minute ducts. The greater vestibular glands may become infected and cause a painful abscess.

Branches of the internal pudendal artery and equivalent veins supply the structures between the labia majora. Each bulb receives an artery to the bulb. The branches anastomose freely to supply the overlying skin and labia minora. Lymph drainage is to iliac nodes.

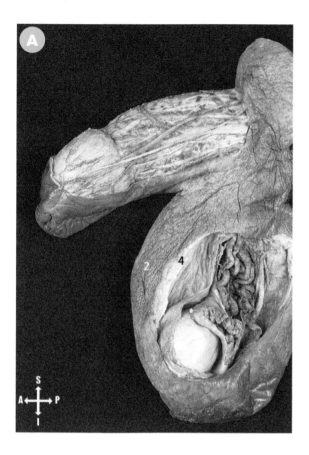

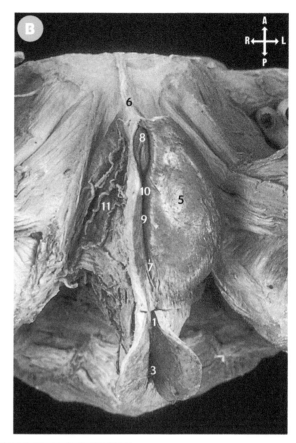

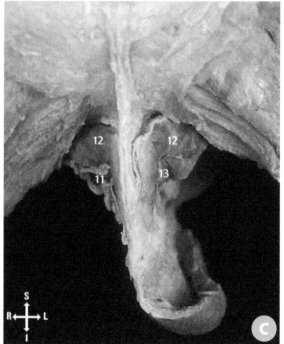

A Left testis, epididymis and penis from the left

B Female perineum from below

C Female perineum from the front

1	Position of perineal body	5	Labium majus, internal surface	9	Vaginal opening	13	Left greater vestibular (Bartholin)
2	Rugose scrotal skin	6	Position of mons pubis overlying	10	Urethral opening		gland (bulb of vestibule dis-
3	Anus		pubic symphysis	11	Bulb of vestibule		sected away)
4	Superficial scrotal (dartos)	7	Posterior commissure	12	Crura of clitoris, fusing to form		
	fascia	8	Prepuce of clitoris		clitoris		

Location of numbers: 1B; 2A; 3B; 4A; 5B; 6B; 7B; 8B; 9B; 10B; 11BC; 12C; 13C.

Penis, clitoris

The penis has three corpora that form its root proximally and its body more distally. The penis transmits the urethra for the passage of urine or semen. Anatomically, the penis is described as if erect.

The corpora cavernosa (1) commence as the two crura, each one attached to the ischiopubic ramus and surrounded by ischiocavernosus muscle (2). Anteriorly, immediately below the pubic symphysis the crura lie side by side, fuse with each other, and pass into the dorsal aspect of the penis. They are tubes, surrounded by thick fascia, the tunica albuginea (3), and full of cavernous tissue that fills with blood to produce erection. Ischiocavernosus, supplied by branches from the perineal branch of the pudendal nerve (S2,3,4) compresses the crus to maintain erection. Each crus receives a deep artery of the penis, from the internal pudendal. The corpora cavernosa communicate with each other across the midline septum (created by their fused fascial sheaths) to enable pressure equalization so that erection is straight.

The corpus spongiosum (4) commences as the bulb of the penis, which is in the midline and attached to the perineal membrane. It receives the urethra (5) and is surrounded by bulbospongiosus muscle (6). The corpus spongiosum continues onto the ventral aspect of the penis and distally it forms the glans penis (7), which is a cap over the two corpora cavernosa. It is a tube of cavernous tissue, but its surrounding fascia is thin, therefore, the internal pressure during erection does not occlude the urethra. The three corpora are surrounded together by a layer of deep fascia, which is itself surrounded by superficial fascia and skin. Proximally the deep fascia is connected to the pubic symphysis by the suspensory ligament of the penis.

The clitoris, like the penis, commences as the crura attached to the ischiopubic rami and covered by ischiocavernosus muscle (8). The crura continue as the corpora cavernosa that meet, fuse and communicate with each other but are only about 2.5 cm long. They are together surrounded by deep fascia and supported by the suspensory ligament (9). But there is no corpus spongiosum and distally the glans of the clitoris is a little isolated cap of erectile tissue, covered by highly sensitive thin skin, and surrounded by the prepuce.

Penile skin is fat free, loose and mobile. Distally it turns inward upon itself and fuses with the rim or corona (10) of the glans to create the foreskin (prepuce) (11). The skin surface inside the prepuce is continuous with that of the glans and the stratified squamous epithelium becomes a mucous membrane. The foreskin must be retractable, otherwise the smegma formed by the desquamation of cells into the space between the foreskin and glans may become infected. A non-retractable prepuce is usually surgically removed (circumcision).

Blood and nerve supply

Blood supply to the penis and clitoris is via branches of the internal pudendal arteries and equivalent veins. A deep artery supplies each crus and corpus cavernosum.

The penis has arteries to the bulb, to supply it, the corpus spongiosum and the glans. There are also dorsal arteries (12), under the deep fascia on the dorsum of the penis to supply the skin, glans and corpora cavernosa. Equivalent veins drain into the prostatic plexus. There is usually a single deep dorsal vein lying within the deep fascia between the dorsal arteries. There is often an additional single or paired superficial dorsal vein (13), outside the deep fascia, on the dorsum of the penis and draining to the external pudendal vein, which is a tributary of the great saphenous.

The clitoris has dorsal arteries that pass on its dorsal surface to supply the glans and prepuce, with the dorsal vein lying between them. (There are not the deep and dorsal veins as in the penis).

Lymph drainage is to the superficial inguinal nodes. Nerve supply to the skin of the proximal penis is via L1, the ilio-inguinal nerve. But the rest is supplied by the dorsal nerve of the penis (14), which is the continuation of the pudendal nerve (S2,3,4). Clitoral nerve supply is via the dorsal nerve of the clitoris and perineal branches of the pudendal nerve. These also carry sympathetic fibres from the pelvic plexus.

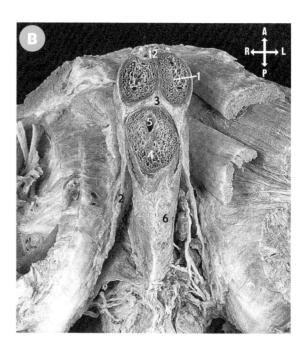

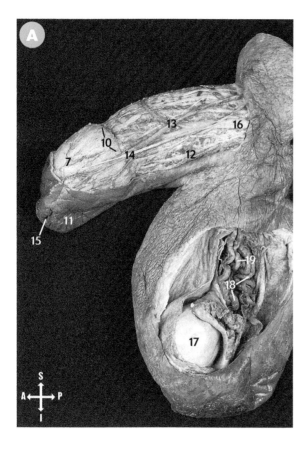

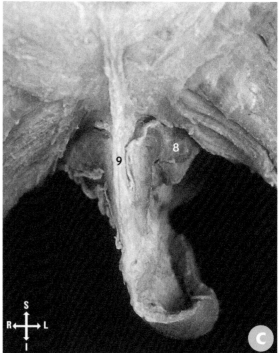

A Left testis, epididymis and penis from the left
B Male perineum from the front
C Female perineum from the front

1	Corpora cavernosa of penis	6	Bulbospongiosus	10	Corona of glans	15	External urethral orifice
2	Ischiocavernosus	7	Glans penis	11	Foreskin (prepuce) of penis	16	Lateral superficial vein
3	Tunica albuginea	8	Crus of clitoris and ischio-	12	Dorsal artery, vein and nerve	17	Testis
4	Corpus spongiosum		cavernosus	13	Superficial dorsal vein	18	Pampiniform venous plexus
5	Urethra	9	Suspensory ligament of clitoris	14	Superficial dorsal nerve	19	Vas (ductus) deferens

Location of numbers: 1B; 2B; 3B; 4B; 5B; 6B; 7A; 8C; 9C; 10A; 11A; 12AB; 13A; 14A; 15A; 16A; 17A; 18A; 19A.

Testes, seminal vesicles, prostate gland

The testes

The testes are the paired oval-shaped male gonads that secrete sex hormones as well as creating sperm. Each testis is surrounded by a tough white fascial coat, the tunica albuginea (1), which facilitates sperm transport by maintaining a slight positive pressure within the testis.

The seminiferous tubules create and transport sperm. They converge into tubules, the rete testis that leads to the head of the epididymis (2) that is applied to the posterior aspect of the testis. The epididymis is a hugely coiled tube for transport and maturation of sperm. It has a head, body (3) and tail (4). At the inferior pole of the testis the tail becomes the vas or ductus deferens that is also convoluted at its commencement.

The vas (ductus) deferens (5) ascends medial to the epididymis, up the posterior aspect of the testis in the spermatic cord, and then through the inguinal canal. It enters the abdomen at the deep inguinal ring, immediately lateral to the inferior epigastric artery and vein (6). It passes inferiorly, onto the lateral pelvic wall and then across the pelvic floor (above the ureter) to meet the duct of the seminal vesicle. Just before doing so it dilates as the ampulla of the vas.

The seminal vesicles

The seminal vesicles (7) lie, one on each side, posterior to the base of the bladder (8), extending laterally posterior to the ureter (9,10). The duct from each vesicle fuses with the vas deferens to create an ejaculatory duct that passes through the prostate gland (11) to enter the urethra. The vesicle is about 5 cm long and secretes seminal fluid, which is slightly alkaline and rich in fructose for nourishment of sperm.

The artery to the vas, from the inferior vesical branch of the internal iliac artery supplies the vas and seminal vesicles. Venous drainage is via the prostatic plexus. The seminal vesicles receive sympathetic innervation from the pelvic plexus and lymph drains to the iliac nodes.

The prostate gland

The prostate gland is normally the size of a chestnut and is conical in shape, with its base related to the trigone of the bladder and its apex piercing the pelvic floor (12). It secretes a watery, slightly acidic and enzyme-rich (acid phosphatase) fluid to facilitate the passage of sperm.

The glandular element of the prostate is within a fibromuscular stroma, and the whole is surrounded by thick pelvic fascia, anchoring the gland to the pelvic floor, and becoming the puboprostatic ligaments that fix the gland to the pubic bone. Posteriorly, the lower rectum (13) is separated from the prostate by the rectovesical fascia (14) (fascia of Denonvilliers) that contains the ampulla of the vas and the medial parts of the seminal vesicles.

The urethra (15) and ejaculatory ducts are said to divide the prostate into lobes, with a median lobe lying between the ejaculatory ducts and the neck of the bladder (16). Prostatic hypertrophy is extremely common with increasing age. The median lobe may push upward into the bladder neck and urethra, possibly disturbing continence, and definitely obstructing urinary flow. Although general prostatic enlargement is palpable by rectal examination, enlargement of this so-called median lobe towards the bladder may not be.

Prostatic branches of the inferior vesical artery supply the prostate. There is a large plexus of veins in its surrounding fascia. These drain to the internal iliac vein. But they also anastomose with veins entering the valveless plexus of internal vertebral veins, facilitating the spread of prostatic tumour to the vertebral column. Lymph drainage is to the iliac nodes. The pelvic plexus provides sympathetic supply.

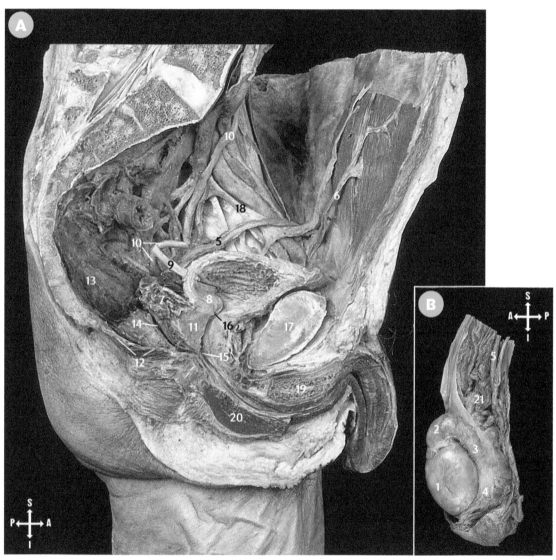

A   Left male pelvic viscera in sagittal section (from the right)
B   Left testicle (from the left)

1	Tunica albuginea around testis	7	Left seminal vesicle	13 Rectum
2	Head of epididymis	8	Base of bladder	14 Rectovesical fascia
3	Body of epididymis	9	Right ureter (distal end)	15 Urethra
4	Tail of epididymis	10	Left ureter	16 Neck of bladder
5	Left vas (ductus) deferens	11	Prostate gland	17 Pubic symphysis
6	Inferior epigastric vessels	12	Cut edge of levator ani	18 Superior vesical artery

19 Corpus cavernosum
20 Bulb of penis
21 Pampiniform venous plexus

Location of numbers: 1B; 2B; 3B; 4B; 5AB; 6A; 7A; 8A; 9A; 10A; 11A; 12A; 13A; 14A; 15A; 16A; 17A; 18A; 19A; 20A; 21B.

Bladder, female urethra, vagina

Bladder

The bladder (1) stores urine and lies anteriorly in the pelvis behind the pubic bones and symphysis (2). It has a triangular base or trigone (3), which in the female lies anterior to the upper vagina (4), uterine cervix (5) and pelvic floor (6). In the male, the trigone lies anterior to the seminal vesicles, rectum and pelvic floor. The ureters (7,8) enter the posterolateral corners of the trigone. The bladder wall is formed by detrusor muscle and lined internally by transitional epithelium, which allows distension. The tone in the detrusor 'pays out' as the bladder fills.

The bladder base and neck (anterior end of trigone) – where the urethra (9) emerges – are fixed to the underlying pelvic structures and pelvic fascia. The latter thickens as pubovesical ligaments. The remainder of the bladder is free to ascend out of the pelvis and into the abdomen (if it contains approximately 500 mL), but always outside the peritoneum (10), immediately posterior to the anterior abdominal wall. The apex is continuous with the obliterated urachus that may be visible as the median umbilical ligament. As the pelvis is a relatively small cavity the bladder is related to its lateral walls (levator ani and obturator internus), the branches of the internal iliac vessels, and the pelvic plexus of nerves.

The bladder is supplied by the superior and inferior vesical branches of the internal iliac artery (11) and drains to the vesical plexus (around its base) that drains to the internal iliac veins. Lymph drainage is to the iliac nodes. The nerve supply is derived from the lumbar splanchnic sympathetic nerves (L1,2) passing in the hypogastric nerves to the pelvic plexus, and from the parasympathetic sacral splanchnics (S2,3,4). Detrusor is controlled by the parasympathetics and the smooth muscle of the trigone and bladder neck by the sympathetics.

Female urethra

The female urethra transmits urine to the exterior. It passes through the pelvic floor to continue in the ante-rior vaginal wall and is a closed slit, 4 cm long. The short urethra predisposes the female to urinary tract infections, although the mucous membrane falls into folds that contact each other. Smooth muscle from the bladder neck descends longitudinally into the urethra to help pull it open during micturition. Other smooth muscle fibres encircle the urethra providing a sphincteric effect. But urinary continence is dependent on pressure from the surrounding pelvic organs on the bladder neck and proximal urethra, before it passes through the pelvic floor. If the bladder drops and the urethra is below the pelvic floor, continence may be compromised.

Vagina

The vagina is a tube passing upward and backward, through the perineum and through the pubovaginalis part of levator ani, to receive the cervix just above the pelvic floor. The anterior and posterior walls are opposed to each other so the vagina is a narrow slit. The wall is of smooth muscle and the mucous membrane (stratified squamous epithelium) is folded so that it may allow distension during intercourse and childbirth.

As the cervix pushes into the vagina, the vaginal wall bulges around it causing small anterior and lateral fornices and a larger posterior fornix. Care must be taken during vaginal hysterectomy to avoid damage to the ureters. The posterior fornix is distensible and may hide foreign bodies. It is also directly related to the peritoneum of the recto-uterine pouch (of Douglas) (17).

Within the urogenital diaphragm the urethra and the vagina are encircled by the striated, external urethral sphincter, whose nerve supply is via perineal branches of the pudendal nerve (S2,3,4). Sensory supply of the urethra and vagina is also via these nerves.

Blood supply to the vagina and urethra is by variable branches from uterine, vaginal and internal pudendal branches of the internal iliac artery. Venous drainage is via the vaginal plexus, draining to the internal iliac veins (20). Lymph drainage from the upper vagina and urethra is to the iliac nodes and from the lower to the superficial inguinal nodes.

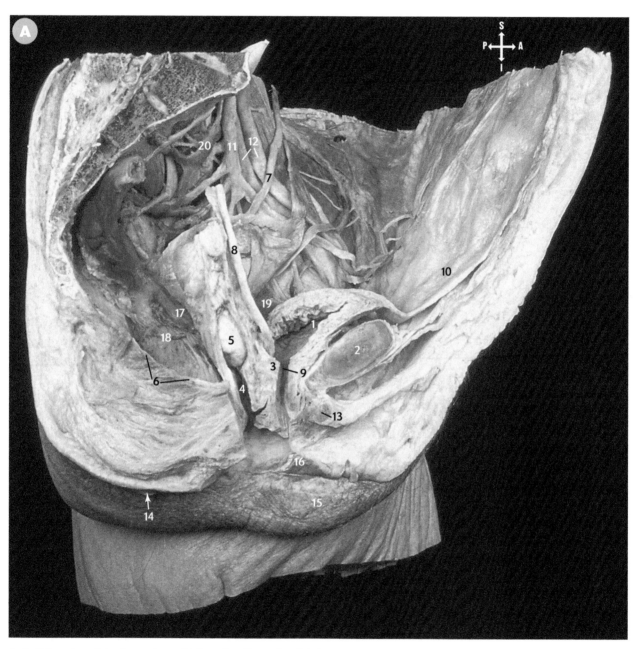

A **Left female pelvic viscera in sagittal section (from the right)**

1 Bladder	6 Cut edge of levator ani	11 Internal iliac artery	16 Labium minus
2 Pubic symphysis	7 Left ureter (displaced anteriorly)	12 External iliac artery and vein	17 Recto-uterine pouch (of Douglas)
3 Base of bladder	8 Right ureter	13 Clitoris	18 Rectum
4 Vagina	9 Urethra	14 Anus	19 Vesico-uterine pouch
5 Cervix of uterus	10 Peritoneum	15 Labium majus	20 Internal iliac vein

Pelvic ureter, male urethra

The ureters

After entering the pelvis the ureters (1,2) lie antero-medial to branches of the internal iliac artery (3). In the female they lie posterior to the ovaries, before passing medially and anteriorly toward the bladder base, inferior to the uterine arteries, just lateral to the vaginal lateral fornices. In the male the vas deferens (4) crosses above and anterior to the ureter. The ureters enter the posterolateral corners of the trigone and pass obliquely through the bladder wall, creating a flap-valve effect, to prevent urinary reflux.

The pelvic part of the ureter picks up its blood supply and innervation from branches of the gonadal and vesical arteries. There is equivalent venous and lymphatic drainage.

Male urethra

The urethra transports urine from the bladder (5) to its slit-like opening on the glans penis (6). As the neck of the bladder (7) opens into the urethra, it is completely surrounded by the prostate gland (8), and together they pass through the puboprostatic part of levator ani (9). The prostate rests on the urogenital diaphragm, but the urethra continues through it.

The urethra is lubricated by mucous glands and also receives the reproductive ducts, prostatic and ejaculatory. It has prostatic (10), membranous (11) and penile (12) parts that in total follow an S-shaped course: vertically downward through the prostate; forward through the membranous part; and eventually downward again in the penile part, when the penis is not erect.

The prostatic urethra has a midline, longitudinal ridge posteriorly, the urethral crest. The groove on each side of this receives the opening of many prostatic ducts. Halfway down the crest there is a small enlargement, the seminal colliculus or verumontanum. Here are the openings of the ejaculatory ducts and the utricle, a functionless embryological remnant. Normally the urethra is closed with its mucous membrane thrown into folds. The muscle of the bladder wall is continuous with the fibromuscular stroma of the prostate gland, and the muscle of the bladder neck continues into the prostatic urethra. Some fibres are longitudinal, but most encircle the proximal urethra as the internal (smooth muscle) urethral sphincter that prevents the backflow of semen into the bladder during ejaculation (see p. 171).

The membranous urethra is the part passing through the urogenital diaphragm that contains the striated muscle of the external urethral sphincter (13), which surrounds the urethra and is supplied by perineal branches of the pudendal nerve (S2,3,4). The urethra passes through the bulb of the penis (14) and then into its corpus spongiosum (15). In the bulb the urethra receives the bulbo-urethral ducts that carry lubricating mucus from the bulbo-urethral glands in the urogenital diaphragm. The bulb itself is surrounded by bulbospongiosus muscle that contracts to expel the last drops of urine or semen.

The urethra reaches the glans, and dilates as the navicular fossa, before narrowing to its external opening. Small mucous glands open into the navicular fossa, and also appear as urethral lacunae along the penile urethra.

The same arteries that supply the prostate and penis supply the urethra (inferior vesical, artery to the bulb, dorsal artery of the penis). Its venous drainage is to the prostatic plexus and internal iliac vein (19). Lymph drainage is to internal iliac nodes. Sensory nerve supply is via the pudendal nerve (S2,3,4).

During urethral catheterization in the male, care must be taken to straighten the curves of the urethra manually. It is possible to rupture the urethra in its thinner membranous part, and also to create false passages through the prostate gland.

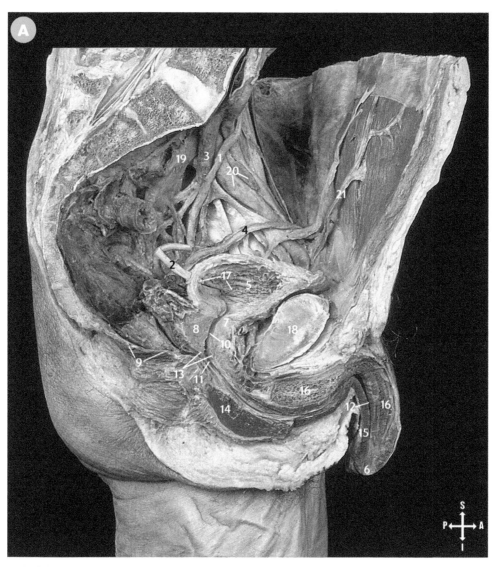

A **Left male pelvic viscera in sagittal section (from the right)**

1	Left ureter	7	Neck of bladder	13	External urethral sphincter	19	Internal iliac vein
2	Right ureter (distal end)	8	Prostate gland	14	Bulb of penis	20	External iliac artery and vein
3	Internal iliac artery	9	Cut edge of levator ani	15	Corpus spongiosum	21	Inferior epigastric vessels
4	Left vas (ductus) deferens	10	Prostatic urethra	16	Corpus cavernosum		
5	Bladder	11	Membranous urethra	17	Ureteric openings		
6	Glans of penis	12	Penile urethra	18	Pubic symphysis		

Rectum, anal canal

Rectum

The rectum (1) lies posteriorly within the pelvic cavity, following the concavity of the sacrum (2). It is the continuation of the sigmoid colon and holds faeces immediately prior to evacuation. It is about 12 cm long, starts at S3, and becomes wider inferiorly, dilating as the rectal ampulla. It takes a sinuous course of left, right, left curves. The sigmoid enters it from the left, creating a concavity to the left at the start of the rectum. The middle concavity is on the opposite side, the right, and there is a smaller, less consistent concavity, again to the left, at the lower end of the rectal ampulla, just above the anorectal junction. At the concavities the rectal wall tends to push into the lumen creating three 'shelves' or rectal valves (of Houston) that may be palpable on rectal examination and visible on proctoscopy and sigmoidoscopy. The middle, right-sided 'shelf' is the most prominent.

As it passes through the puborectalis part of levator ani (3) it turns sharply downward and backward as the 4 cm long anal canal (4), which is for the evacuation of faeces.

Anal canal

The anal canal, which is entirely in the perineum, has its mucous membrane raised into between five and ten anal columns (of Morgagni) by the underlying terminal branches of the superior rectal artery and vein. These columns end about half-way down the canal, and folds of epithelium, the anal valves, link their lower ends. The lubricating, anal mucous glands open into the anal sinuses between the columns, above and behind the anal valves. Following years of wear and tear, these features may be difficult to distinguish in the elderly.

The line of anal valves is the dentate or pectinate line, and it represents the change in embryological development from entoderm to ectoderm. There are other significant changes at the pectinate line. Above it, the mucous membrane is columnar and below it is stratified squamous. Above the line the innervation is

autonomic, sensitive to distension but not to pain, and able to distinguish between flatus and faeces. Below the line the innervation is somatic and the anal canal is sensitive to painful stimuli, such as ulceration, fissures or injections.

For about 1.5 cm below the pectinate line the thin stratified squamous epithelium covers the pecten that ends at an indistinct white line which overlies the intersphincteric groove, where the internal anal sphincter ends. At the white line the stratified squamous epithelium begins to develop the features of skin (sweat glands, keratinization, hair follicles) and soon becomes the anus. During defecation the anal canal opens and everts onto the surface as far as the pecten.

The mucous membrane of the anal canal is folded to allow distension during defecation. On proctoscopy it bulges into the proctoscope as anal cushions, usually at the positions of three, seven and eleven on a clock face. In a similar way the mucous membrane may bulge (possibly caused by distended submucosal veins) into and down the anal canal, as piles or haemorrhoids, which may remain outside the anus. Bleeding from the capillaries of this mucous membrane is known as bleeding haemorrhoids.

Blood supply to the rectum and anal canal is via the superior rectal branches of the inferior mesenteric artery, the variable middle rectal branch of the internal iliac (8), and the inferior rectal branch of the internal pudendal. There is free anastomosis between all these vessels. The venous drainage is via a similar route, returning via the superior rectal veins, to inferior mesenteric and portal vein or via the internal iliac vein (10) (portosystemic anastomosis).

Lymph drainage is to the sacral and iliac nodes, but the upper rectum drains to the inferior mesenteric nodes, and the lower anal canal to the superficial inguinal nodes. Innervation is via the autonomic system or via the inferior rectal branch of the pudendal nerve. Parasympathetic afferents return to S2–S4, from which the pudendal nerve arises, allowing the important reflexes between the autonomic and somatic systems (see p. 170).

During rectal (digital) examination in the male the prostate gland (11) can be assessed, but the seminal vesicles (15) are only palpable if they are abnormal.

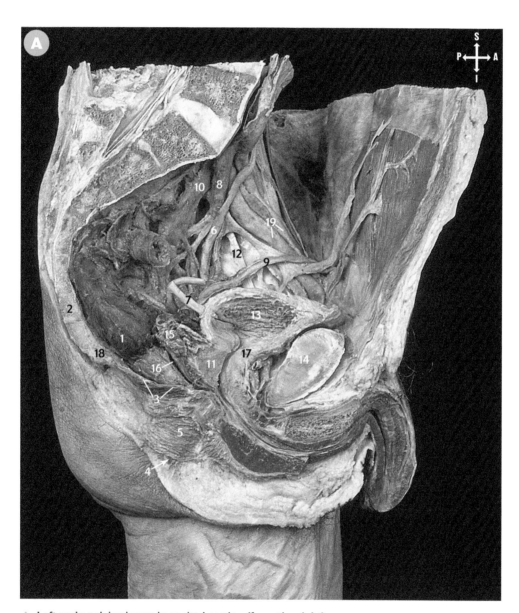

A **Left male pelvic viscera in sagittal section (from the right)**

1	Rectum	6	Left ureter	11	Prostate gland	16	Rectovesical fascia
2	Sacrum	7	Right ureter (distal end)	12	Obturator nerve	17	Neck of bladder
3	Cut edge of levator ani	8	Internal iliac artery	13	Bladder	18	Coccyx
4	Anus (lower end of anal canal)	9	Left vas (ductus) deferens	14	Pubic symphysis	19	External iliac artery and vein
5	External anal sphincter	10	Internal iliac vein	15	Left seminal vesicle		

■ Ovary, uterine tubes

Ovary

During reproductive life, under the control of the pituitary gland, the ovary (1) secretes the female sex hormones, oestrogen and progesterone, as well as monthly, the ovum.

In the adult female, the ovary is oval in shape and about the size of the terminal phalanx of the thumb. It is suspended by a short mesovarium from the posterior leaf of the broad ligament (2), and lies in a fossa on the lateral pelvic wall with the ureter (4) posteriorly and the obturator nerve laterally. Consequently, great care must be taken during ovarian surgery to avoid damaging the ureter. Inflammatory conditions of the ovary may irritate the obturator nerve and cause pain to be referred to the medial thigh. In elderly women the ovary is usually shrunken. During pregnancy it is lifted out of the pelvis and may return to lie in variable positions within the pelvis.

The ovary brings its blood and nerve supply with it from its initial position on the posterior abdominal wall. The ovarian artery (5) leaves the aorta at the level of L2, passes down the posterior abdominal wall and into the suspensory ligament of the ovary (6), before reaching the ovary in its mesovarium. Venous drainage is via a plexus of veins that accompany the artery and eventually coalesce to form the ovarian vein. The right ovarian vein drains to the inferior vena cava, the left ovarian vein to the left renal vein. Lymph drainage is to the para-aortic nodes.

Sympathetic innervation, with its accompanying afferents, is derived from the lesser splanchnic nerves (T10,11). Therefore, ovarian (visceral) pain may refer to the T10,11 dermatomes, in the midline, the peri-umbilical region (as well as to the medial thigh via the obturator nerve).

During development, the peritoneum overlying the ovary is said to become incorporated into its wall, therefore, the ovary is the only truly intraperitoneal structure. At ovulation the ovum is secreted into the peritoneal cavity, to be 'picked up' by the uterine tube. Rarely, but dangerously, it is possible for the ovum to be fertilized, and then implant and develop as an ectopic pregnancy in the peritoneal cavity (see pp. 169 and 170).

Uterine (Fallopian) tubes

The uterine tubes (7) emerge from each side of the uterus to lie in the upper free edge of the broad ligament. The part of the broad ligament that acts as a mesentery for the tube is called the mesosalpinx. Sperm entering the vagina pass through the cavity of the uterus and into the uterine tube, where fertilization of the ovum occurs. The fertilized ovum is then transported down the tube to implant and develop within the uterus. Should such transport not occur the fertilized ovum might develop in the tube as an ectopic, tubal pregnancy.

Medially, the uterine tube has an intramural part, within the wall of the uterus. Moving laterally it has an isthmus, ampulla, infundibulum (8), and finally a splayed, fimbriated end (9). The infundibulum pierces the posterior leaf of the broad ligament so that the fimbriae overhang the ovary in the peritoneal cavity. One fimbria usually attaches to the ovary.

The tube receives blood supply via an anastomosis between the ovarian and uterine arteries. Venous drainage is to the ovarian and uterine veins. Lymph drainage is to the para-aortic nodes.

The afferent nerve supply returns to the T11,12 and L1 segments of the cord. Consequently, tubal pain is lower abdominal but may extend to the iliac fossa and, if on the right, may confuse the diagnosis of appendicitis.

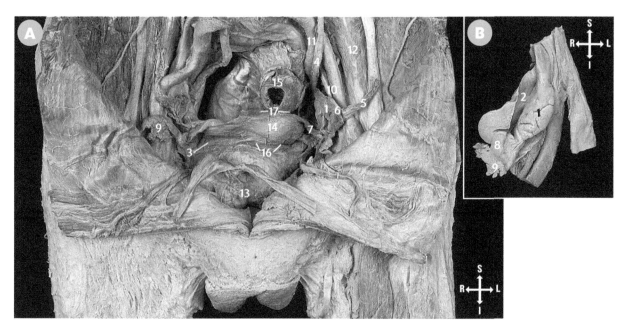

A Female pelvic contents (from the front)
B Left ovary (from behind)

1	Ovary	6	Suspensory ligament of ovary	11	Internal iliac artery	16	Vesico-uterine pouch
2	Posterior leaf of broad ligament	7	Uterine tube	12	Psoas major	17	Recto-uterine pouch (of Douglas)
3	Anterior leaf of broad ligament	8	Infundibulum of uterine tube	13	Bladder		
4	Left ureter	9	Fimbriated end of uterine tube	14	Fundus of uterus		
5	Ovarian artery	10	External iliac artery and vein	15	Rectum		

Location of numbers: 1AB; 2B; 3A; 4A; 5A; 6A; 7A; 8B; 9AB; 10A; 11A; 12A; 13A; 14A; 15A; 16A; 17A.

Uterus, cervix

Uterus

The uterus (1) is a single organ in the midline (or slightly deviated from it) of the female pelvis. Its cavity is for the implantation and development of the embryo and its placenta. Normally the uterus is about the size and shape of a medium pear, but during pregnancy it hugely increases in size. It has a fundus (above the entry of the uterine tubes), a body and a cervix.

The uterine wall is muscular so that it can relax and expand during pregnancy but contract during labour. The mucous lining (endometrium) is controlled by the cyclical ovarian hormones, the mucosa being prepared each month for implantation of the fertilized ovum but shed at menstruation if that does not occur.

Cervix

The cervix (2) is a small cylinder with a very narrow lumen that is effectively occluded by its interdigitating folds of mucous membrane. Motile sperm swim their way through. The cervix pushes into the anterior wall of the vagina, therefore has vaginal and supravaginal parts. Normally it meets the vagina (3) at right angles, the anteverted position. Where the body of the uterus and the cervix meet, the body is tilted forward in the anteflexed position. This combination of anteversion and anteflexion means the uterus has an antero-inferior surface related to the bladder and a postero-superior surface related to coils of intestine. The cervix and vagina meet each other low down in the pelvic cavity, just superior to the pelvic floor (4) and in front of the rectum (5). Cervical dilatation during the early stages of labour may be assessed by rectal examination.

It is important that the uterus is maintained in its normal anatomical position and there are a multitude of factors to uterine support. The surrounding organs, all closely fitted into the pelvic cavity, support each other. The muscular pelvic floor and the integrity of the perineal body (6) are essential. The pelvic floor fascia thickens around the uterine arteries as lateral ligaments. Other fascial thickenings pass from the uterus to the sacrum (uterosacral) and from the cervix to the pubis (pubocervical). The broad (8) and round (9) ligaments maintain anteversion and anteflexion.

Repeated pregnancy may weaken the supports allowing 'slippage' of the uterus and vagina. This may well alter the position of the bladder to cause poor urinary control, stress or urge incontinence and urinary infections. In more extreme situations rectal continence may be affected, and the uterus may prolapse into the vagina and even descend to appear externally. Disruption of anteversion and anteflexion may cause backache and difficulty in conception.

The uterus is supplied by the uterine arteries, which are branches of the internal iliac arteries (10). These anastomose freely with each other and with the ovarian arteries, which tend to supply the fundus. Consequently, venous drainage is mainly to the internal iliac veins (13), but to the ovarian veins (14) as well. As the uterine arteries pass along the pelvic floor to the lateral aspect of the uterus, they pass above the ureter (15,16), just lateral to the cervix and the lateral vaginal fornices. During surgery great care must be taken not to damage the ureter.

Lymph drainage of the fundus tends to follow the ovarian artery to the para-aortic nodes. But the body and cervix drain to sacral and iliac nodes, usually the external iliac. Some lymph drainage may follow the round ligament to the superficial inguinal nodes.

Nerve supply is via the pelvic plexus containing both sympathetic (T10–12 and L1) and parasympathetic (S2–4) components. Afferents from the body and fundus are thought to pass with the sympathetics so that pain is lower abdominal. But those of the cervix are thought to pass with the parasympathetics giving rise to deep pelvic pain.

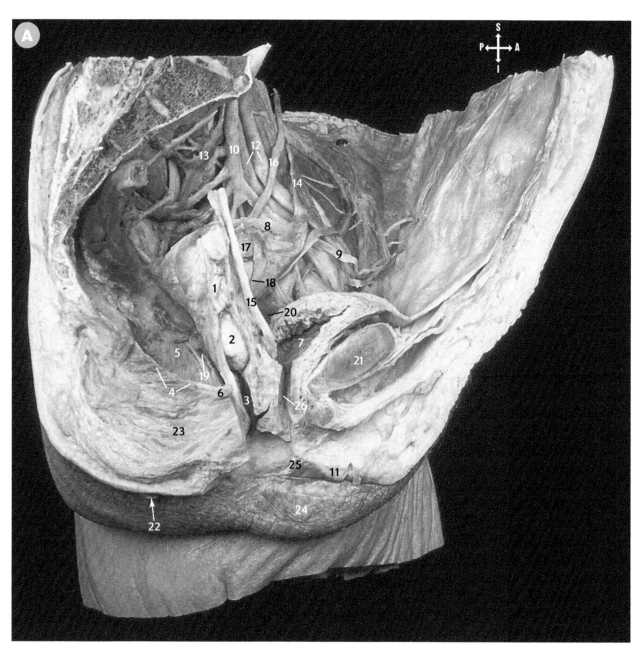

A Left female pelvic viscera in sagittal section (from the right)

1	Body of uterus	7	Bladder	15	Right ureter	23	External anal sphincter
2	Cervix of uterus	8	Broad ligament	16	Left ureter	24	Labium majus
3	Vagina	9	Round ligament	17	Ovary	25	Labium minus
4	Cut edge of levator ani (pelvic floor)	10	Internal iliac artery	18	Uterine (Fallopian) tube	26	Urethra
5	Rectum	11	Clitoris	19	Recto-uterine pouch (of Douglas)		
6	Perineal body (central perineal tendon)	12	External iliac artery and vein	20	Vesico-uterine pouch		
		13	Internal iliac vein	21	Pubic symphysis		
		14	Ovarian artery and vein	22	Anus		

Part VII

The Torso

The torso

Upper body and thorax

Any movement at the shoulder joint is accompanied by movements of the pectoral girdle (scapula and clavicle). Muscles arise from the torso and skull to attach to the clavicle (1), scapula and humerus. The scapula may be:

- rotated upward during abduction by trapezius (2), serratus anterior (3)
- rotated downward during adduction by pectoralis major (4,5) and minor (9), latissimus dorsi (10)
- protracted by pectoralis major and minor, serratus anterior
- retracted by rhomboids (11), trapezius, levator scapulae.

The muscles combine to brace the scapula against the thoracic wall and hold its position to provide a platform for the upper limb when carrying weights or pushing. Many are accessory muscles of respiration. Anterior muscles that attach to the humerus flex the shoulder joint, posterior muscles extend it.

- Trapezius (accessory (XI)) – from skull, cervical spines via ligamentum nuchae and thoracic spines to scapular spine, acromion process, and lateral one-third of clavicle (posterior aspect).

- Serratus anterior (long thoracic (C5,6,7)) – from upper eight ribs to medial border and inferior angle of scapula. Injury to the long thoracic nerve allows 'winging' of the scapula and full arm abduction as in brushing one's hair is difficult.
- Pectoralis major (pectoral (C5–8)) – from manubrium, sternum, upper six costal cartilages, and medial clavicle to anterior lip of intertubercular groove of humerus.
- Pectoralis minor (pectoral (C5–8)) – from the third, fourth and fifth ribs to coracoid process of scapula.
- Latissimus dorsi (thoracodorsal (C6,7,8)) – from ilium, thoracolumbar fascia (12), lower four ribs and inferior angle of scapula to floor of intertubercular groove, after winding around teres major (13).
- Rhomboid major and minor (dorsal scapular C 5) – from the spines of C7–T5 to medial border of scapula.

- The triangle of auscultation (14) is between the scapula, trapezius and latissimus dorsi.
- Deltoid (15) (axillary (C5,6)) – from scapular spine, acromion process and lateral one-third clavicle (anterior aspect) to mid-shaft humerus, lateral aspect. Muscle fibres lie anterior to, posterior to, and over the shoulder joint. Therefore, deltoid flexes, extends and abducts.

Abdomen

Muscles of the abdominal wall support the abdominal contents and the vertebral column.

Rectus abdominis (16) (segmental T7–12) flexes the trunk. It lies on either side adjacent to the midline. It passes from the costal cartilages of the fifth to seventh ribs to the pubic crest (17) and symphysis (18). It is partially divided by three transverse tendinous intersections (19). On a slim subject the muscle in between the intersections may form visible bulges on the anterior abdomen.

Each rectus abdominis lies within a rectus sheath (20) created by the aponeuroses of external oblique (21), internal oblique and transversus abdominis. The tendinous intersections fuse with the anterior layer of the sheath, but not its posterior layer. External oblique is superficial, therefore forms the anterior layer of the sheath. The aponeurosis of internal oblique (the deeper muscle layer) splits to enclose rectus abdominis, contributing to both the anterior and posterior layers of the sheath. Transversus abdominis is the deepest layer and its aponeurosis forms the posterior layer of the sheath.

At a variable distance, but usually just a few centimetres below the umbilicus, the posterior rectus sheath stops and all the aponeuroses pass anterior to rectus abdominis. The end of the posterior sheath is the arcuate line (of Douglas) and the inferior epigastric artery and vein enter the sheath here.

In the midline these aponeuroses all fuse to form the relatively avascular linea alba (22). Its position is seen as the vertical midline groove in the living abdomen. The lateral edge of rectus abdominis is visible as the linea semilunaris. The umbilicus (25), in the midline, lies opposite L3/L4 in a slim, fit subject, but indicates the T10,11 dermatomes.

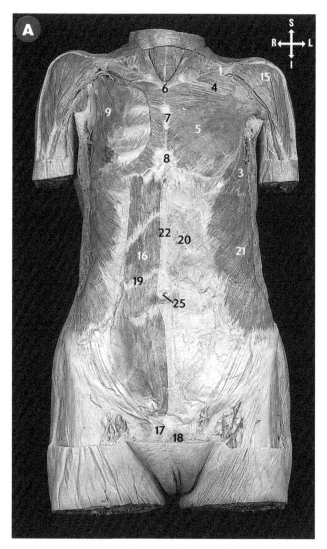

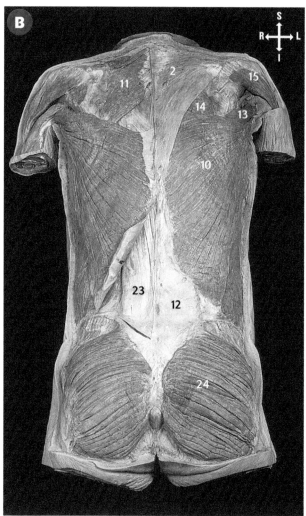

A Anterior muscles of the torso (from the front)
B Posterior muscles of the torso (from behind)

1	Clavicle	6	Manubrium	13	Teres major	20	Rectus sheath

1 Clavicle
2 Trapezius
3 Serratus anterior
4 Clavicular part of pectoralis major
5 Sternocostal part of pectoralis major

6 Manubrium
7 Body of sternum
8 Xiphoid process
9 Pectoralis minor
10 Latissimus dorsi
11 Rhomboids (major and minor)
12 Thoracolumbar fascia

13 Teres major
14 Triangle of auscultation
15 Deltoid
16 Rectus abdominis
17 Position of pubic crest
18 Pubic symphysis
19 Tendinous intersection

20 Rectus sheath
21 External oblique
22 Linea alba
23 Erector spinae
24 Gluteus maximus
25 Umbilicus

Location of numbers: 1A; 2B; 3A; 4A; 5A; 6A; 7A; 8A; 9A; 10B; 11B; 12B; 13B; 14B; 15AB; 16A; 17A; 18A; 19A; 20A; 21A; 22A; 23B; 24B; 25A.

Part VIII

The Upper Limb

Axilla, upper limb fascia, veins, arteries

Axilla

The axilla is inferior to the shoulder joint and filled with fat, lymph nodes and the neurovascular supply for the upper limb. Its apex is bounded by the first rib, scapula and clavicle (1), and through it structures pass between the root of the neck and the upper limb. Serratus anterior (5), the ribs and intercostal muscles lie medially. The intertubercular groove of the humerus lies laterally. Subscapularis forms the posterior wall. Immediately inferior to it, latissimus dorsi (6) and teres major are palpable as the posterior axillary fold. Pectoralis major (7,8) and minor (9) form the anterior wall, with the inferior edge of major palpable as the anterior axillary fold. The axillary lymph nodes (12) drain the upper limb, but more importantly in the female, they drain much of the breast. The nodes are arranged as follows:

- A – anterior (pectoral) behind pectoralis minor, draining breast and anterior body wall above umbilicus
- P – posterior (subscapular) on subscapularis, draining posterior body wall above umbilicus
- I – infraclavicular
- C – central
- A – apical
- L – lateral, around axillary vein, draining upper limb. The anterior, posterior and lateral groups drain to the central group that, along with the infraclavicular group, drains to the apical nodes. Afferents from the latter communicate with the deep cervical nodes and drain to the subclavian lymph trunk. Individual groups are usually indistinguishable in a normal cadaveric dis-

section. But they are significant in staging the spread of breast tumours. The communication between axillary and deep cervical lymph nodes means that breast tumours may spread to the latter.

Upper limb fascia

The upper limb has a thin sleeve of deep fascia (13) that attaches to palpable bony prominences (spine of scapula, acromion, clavicle, humeral epicondyles and subcutaneous border of ulna). It gives origin to muscles and sends septa between muscle groups to form compartments in which the muscles move in relation to each other and to the overlying skin. The compartments may limit swelling following crush injuries or fractures. The resultant pressure (compartment syndrome) may compress the nerves and blood vessels within the compartments and cause muscle ischaemia with consequent necrosis and (Volkmann's) contracture. Distally the fascia specializes as extensor and flexor retinacula (14), and the palmar aponeurosis (15).

Veins

The veins have valves to prevent backflow. The deep veins commence as venae comitantes of the arteries, but converge on the axillary vein (16), as do the superficial veins. The veins draining the fingers and hand pass dorsally to form the dorsal carpal plexus, which laterally becomes the cephalic vein (17) and medially the basilic vein. Both are visible under the skin, along with many other, variable veins.

The cephalic vein passes proximally up the radial border of the forearm to the elbow, then lateral to biceps (18) before running in the groove between pectoralis major and deltoid (22). At the upper end of this groove it pierces the fascia to enter the axillary vein. At the wrist, the cephalic is in a constant position and may be used as a site of 'cutting down' through the skin to locate the vein for emergency, rapid access.

The basilic vein passes proximally on the ulnar border of the forearm to the elbow, and then medial to biceps before piercing the deep fascia half way up the arm to join the venae comitantes of the brachial artery and become the axillary vein. Anterior to the elbow the cephalic and basilic veins are connected by the median cubital vein (23), passing medially and superiorly. It usually receives the median vein of the forearm and lies anterior to the brachial artery (24) and median nerve (25), but separated from them by the bicipital aponeurosis (26).

Arteries

Arteries are palpable as pulses when they lie superficially, but may also be compressed against bone. Medial to the tendon of biceps the brachial pulse is palpable at the extended elbow. Proximal to the base of the thumb, lateral to flexor carpi radialis (29), the radial pulse (30) is palpable at the wrist. Arterial variation is common and the brachial artery or its branches may take a course superficial to the aponeurosis.

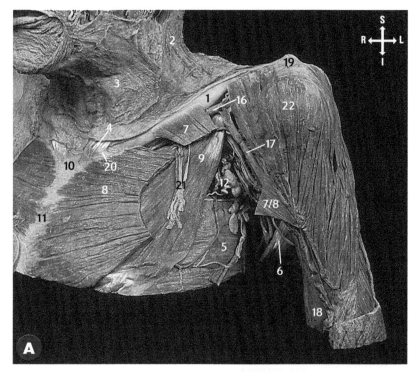

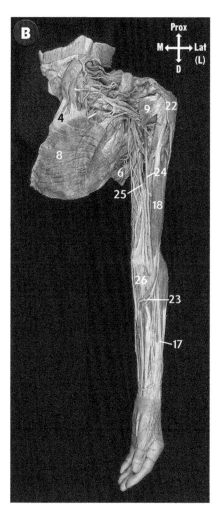

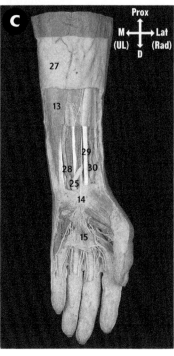

A Left shoulder, superficial structures
   (from the left)
B Left upper limb, superficial structures
   (from the front)
C Left forearm and hand, superficial
   structures (from the front)

1	Clavicle	**8**	Sternocostal part of pectoralis	**16** Axillary vein	**24** Brachial artery
2	Investing layer of deep cervical		major	**17** Cephalic vein	**25** Median nerve
	fascia	**9**	Pectoralis minor	**18** Biceps	**26** Bicipital aponeurosis
3	Platysma	**10**	Manubrium	**19** Acromioclavicular joint	**27** Superficial subcutaneous tissue
4	Sternal head of	**11**	Sternum	**20** Sternoclavicular joint	**28** Ulnar artery
	sternocleidomastoid	**12**	Axillary lymph nodes	**21** Thoraco-acromial vessels and	**29** Flexor carpi radialis
5	Serratus anterior	**13**	Deep fascia of forearm	lateral pectoral nerve	**30** Radial artery
6	Latissimus dorsi	**14**	Flexor retinaculum	**22** Deltoid	
7	Clavicular part of pectoralis major	**15**	Palmar aponeurosis	**23** Median cubital vein	

Location of numbers: **1**A; **2**A; **3**A; **4**AB; **5**A; **6**AB; **7**A; **8**AB; **9**AB; **10**A; **11**A; **12**A; **13**C; **14**C; **15**C; **16**A; **17**AB; **18**AB; **19**A; **20**A; **21**A; **22**AB; **23**B; **24**B;
25BC; **26**B; **27**C; **28**C; **29**C; **30**C.

Shoulder (glenohumeral) joint

Any movement at the shoulder joint is accompanied by movements of the pectoral girdle. (See section on torso, p. 128).

The shoulder is a typical synovial, ball and socket joint between the scapular **glenoid fossa (2)** and the relatively larger **humeral head (3)**. The fibrocartilaginous **glenoid labrum (4)** deepens the fossa. The joint capsule is lax, sacrificing stability for mobility. It attaches to the scapula and glenoid labrum, and to the anatomical neck of the humerus. Medially the capsule dips down the shaft of the humerus to provide extra space for the humeral head during abduction. It maybe minimally strengthened by glenohumeral ligaments anteriorly and a coracohumeral ligament superiorly.

To provide support and stability, the acromial and coracoid processes overhang the joint, as does the coraco-acromial ligament that connects the two processes. The tendon of the long head of biceps lies within the shoulder joint and attaches to the supraglenoid tubercle of the scapula, immediately above the glenoid fossa. The **long head of triceps (6)** attaches to the infraglenoid tubercle, immediately inferior to the fossa, and provides some support for the joint inferiorly. The bones are held in close apposition by surface tension within the joint. But most of the stability is dependent on the musculotendinous, rotator cuff formed by four muscles arising from the scapula and inserting into the humerus, very close to its head, and into the shoulder joint capsule itself. By virtue of their dual insertions they stabilize the shoulder joint, holding the humeral head against the glenoid.

Shoulder movements

- Abduction – **supraspinatus (7)** (suprascapular nerve (C5,6)) passes from the supraspinous fossa of the scapula to the upper facet on the **greater tuberosity of the humerus (8)**. Passing above the joint it initiates abduction.
- External (lateral) rotation – infraspinatus (suprascapular nerve (C5,6)) arises from the posterior aspect of the scapula. **Teres minor (9)** (**axillary nerve (10)** (C5,6)) arises from the lateral border of

the scapula. Both muscles pass posterior to the joint (to the greater tuberosity) therefore must externally rotate it.
- Internal (medial) rotation – **subscapularis (12)** (nerves to subscapularis (C5,6,7) from the posterior cord of the brachial plexus) passes from the anterior aspect of the scapula to the lesser tuberosity of the humerus. As it lies anterior to the joint it must internally rotate it.
- Adduction – **teres major (13)** (lower subscapular nerve (C6,7)) is not part of the musculotendinous cuff as it passes from the inferior angle of the scapula to the posterior lip of the intertubercular groove. It adducts the humerus and as its insertion is in a plane anterior to the shoulder joint it also internally rotates it.

The shoulder joint is a common cause of complaint. Supraspinatus tendon passes in the coraco-acromial bursa, between the upper aspect of the joint capsule and the coraco-acromial ligament. The tendon may become inflamed causing pain during the phase of abduction where it passes beneath the ligament. The tendon may rupture. Subscapularis and infraspinatus also have bursae between their tendons and the joint capsule. All three bursae may communicate with the joint and all three may become painfully inflamed.

The shoulder is weakest at its inferior aspect. Excessive, forced abduction may cause the humeral head to dislocate antero-inferiorly, where it may impinge on the axillary nerve (C5,6) as it winds, with the **posterior circumflex vessels (14)**, around the surgical neck of the humerus, immediately inferior to the joint. Such damage may cause paralysis of **deltoid (15)** and of teres minor. But the important test is for sensory loss over the skin of the lateral arm, the 'regimental patch'. The axillary nerve is also at risk in fractures of the surgical neck of the humerus. The brachial plexus passes from the neck to the upper limb, behind the clavicle. Shoulder dislocation may cause traction injury to the plexus.

To prevent vascular obstruction during joint movements, the arteries proximal to, and distal to joints send branches that anastomose with each other and provide collateral circulations. At the shoulder, there is a rich scapular anastomosis between branches of the subclavian and axillary arteries.

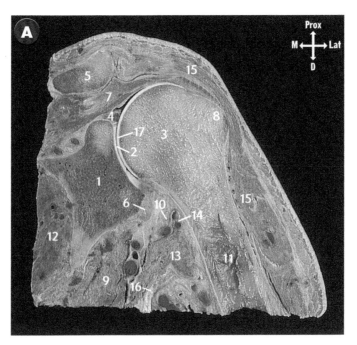

A Coronal section through the left shoulder joint (from the front)

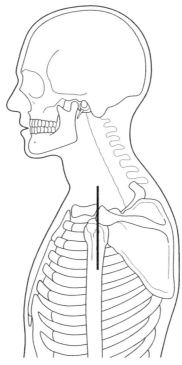

Line diagram adapted from Ellis H, Logan BM, Dixon AK (2001) *Human Sectional Anatomy*. London: Arnold.

1 Scapula	**6** Long head of triceps	**11** Shaft of humerus	**15** Deltoid
2 Glenoid fossa of scapula	**7** Supraspinatus	**12** Subscapularis	**16** Tendon of latissimus dorsi
3 Head of humerus	**8** Greater tuberosity of humerus	**13** Teres major	**17** Cavity of shoulder joint
4 Glenoid labrum	**9** Teres minor	**14** Posterior circumflex artery and	
5 Clavicle	**10** Axillary nerve	vein	

Elbow, superior radio-ulnar, inferior radio-ulnar, wrist and mid-carpal joints

Elbow and superior radio-ulnar joint

The elbow and superior radio-ulnar joints may be considered as one, as they share the same fibrous and synovial joint capsules. Movements of the joint are flexion and extension, plus pronation and supination as the radius rotates around the ulna.

The radius and ulna are held together by the interosseous membrane. The concave radial head (1) lies against the capitulum of the humerus (2), and is clasped to the ulna (3) by the anular ligament (4). The olecranon and coronoid processes of the ulna form a hook that hangs onto the olecranon fossa, trochlear surface (5) and coronoid fossa of the humerus.

The fibrous joint capsule is lax anteriorly and posteriorly to allow flexion and extension, and it attaches at the articular margins of the humerus and ulna. It does not attach to the radius but to the anular ligament. The olecranon, coronoid and radial fossae are included within the capsule so that the equivalent processes of the ulna and radius may enter the fossae during appropriate movements. Each fossa has a small pad of fat between the bone and the synovial membrane.

The capsule is thickened by collateral ligaments. The lateral collateral ligament runs from the lateral humeral epicondyle to the anular ligament and the medial collateral ligament is a triangular ligament with its apex at the medial epicondyle (6), and diverging to the coronoid and olecranon processes of the ulna. The capsule may be pulled out of the way during elbow flexion by a few fibres of brachialis anteriorly, and during extension by triceps posteriorly. There is a subcutaneous bursa over the olecranon as well as bursae superficial to, and deep to the triceps tendon. These bursae may become inflamed, as may the tendinous origins at the medial and lateral epicondyles (the common flexor and common extensor origins).

The median nerve and brachial artery lie anterior to brachialis, itself anterior to the elbow. The ulnar nerve (7) lies posterior to the medial epicondyle. The radial nerve lies deep to brachioradialis (8), lateral to the joint. All these structures are at risk of injury in fractures and dislocations of the elbow. The radial head may accidentally be pulled out of the anular ligament, this usually occurs when children are swung around by their arms.

Inferior radio-ulnar joint

The inferior radio-ulnar joint (13), is supported by the interosseous membrane and by a triangular fibrocartilage disc (14) with its apex attached to the ulnar styloid, and its base attached to the radius (15). Consequently the disc, which moves with the radius in pronation and supination, overlies the head of the ulna (16), preventing the ulna from taking part in the wrist joint.

Wrist joint

The wrist joint itself is between the scaphoid (17), lunate (18) and radius. The hand is carried with the radius during pronation and supination. Forces passing through the hand are transmitted mainly via the scaphoid to the radius. The wrist may flex or extend and deviate in radial or ulnar directions. These movements involve adjunct movements at the mid-carpal joint, between the proximal and distal rows of carpal bones. Although both joints are involved, extension is primarily a wrist joint movement whereas flexion is primarily at the mid-carpal joint.

Distally, the radius, ulna and carpal bones are bound together by a fibrous capsule, strengthened by many ligaments, named by their position and by the bones to which they attach. A fall on the outstretched hand, in a younger person usually causes fracture of the scaphoid with tenderness in the anatomical snuffbox (26). Blood supply to the scaphoid passes from distal to proximal. An undiagnosed/untreated scaphoid fracture may lead to avascular necrosis of the proximal fragment, and consequent early onset of wrist arthritis. A fall on the outstretched hand in an elderly person is more likely to cause a Colles' fracture at the lower end of the radius.

A Coronal section through the left elbow joint (from the front)
B Coronal section through the left hand and wrist joint (from behind)

C Sagittal section through the joints of the left wrist and middle finger (from the left)

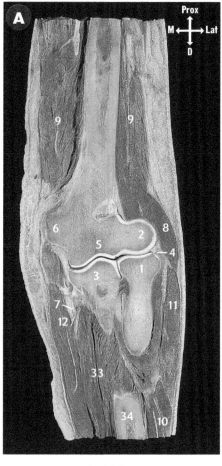

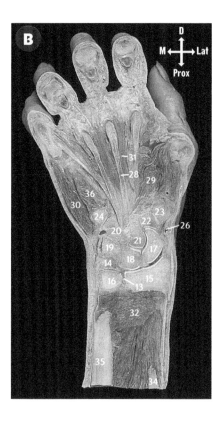

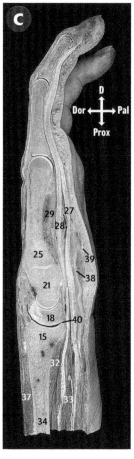

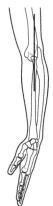

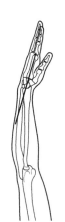

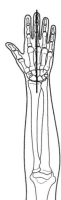

Line diagrams adapted from Ellis H, Logan BM, Dixon AK (2001) *Human Sectional Anatomy*. London: Arnold.

1 Head of radius	**13** Inferior radio-ulnar joint
2 Capitulum of humerus	**14** Articular disc (triangular fibrocartilaginous complex (TFCC))
3 Coronoid process of ulna	
4 Anular ligament	**15** Distal end of radius
5 Trochlea of humerus	**16** Head of ulna
6 Medial epicondyle of humerus	**17** Scaphoid
7 Ulnar nerve	**18** Lunate
8 Brachioradialis	**19** Triquetral
9 Medial head of triceps	**20** Hamate
10 Extensor carpi radialis brevis	**21** Capitate
11 Extensor carpi radialis longus	**22** Trapezoid
12 Flexor carpi ulnaris	

23 Trapezium	**32** Pronator quadratus
24 Base of fifth metacarpal bone	**33** Flexor digitorum profundus
25 Third metacarpal bone	**34** Shaft of radius
26 Radial artery in anatomical snuffbox	**35** Shaft of ulna
	36 Flexor digiti minimi brevis
27 Tendon of flexor digitorum superficialis	**37** Extensor digitorum
	38 Flexor retinaculum
28 Tendon of flexor digitorum profundus	**39** Palmar aponeurosis
	40 Capsule of wrist joint
29 Adductor pollicis	
30 Abductor digiti minimi	
31 Second lumbrical	

Location of numbers: 1A; **2**A; **3**A; **4**A; **5**A; **6**A; **7**A; **8**A; **9**A; **10**A; **11**A; **12**A; **13**B; **14**B; **15**BC; **16**B; **17**B; **18**BC; **19**B; **20**B; **21**BC; **22**B; **23**B; **24**B; **25**C; **26**B; **27**C; **28**BC; **29**BC; **30**B; **31**B; **32**BC; **33**AC; **34**ABC; **35**B; **36**B; **37**C; **38**C; **39**C; **40**C.

Upper limb: anterior muscle groups

Elbow flexion and supination

The anterior compartment of the arm has coraco-brachialis (4), a shoulder adductor, medially with brachialis and biceps anteriorly. Brachialis passes from the humerus to the ulna and flexes the elbow. Biceps (5) has a short head (6) from the coracoid process and a long head (7) from the supraglenoid tubercle of the scapula. Both heads converge on a tendon (8) that inserts into the radial (bicipital) tuberosity, and also into the bicipital aponeurosis (9), which merges with the deep fascia to attach to the ulna. Biceps is a powerful flexor and supinator. The musculocutaneous nerve (11) (C5,6,7) supplies all three muscles before becoming the lateral cutaneous nerve of the forearm.

In the forearm, the muscles are divided into deep and superficial groups. Their actions are: pronation; wrist (carpal) flexion, including radial or ulnar deviation; finger flexion; thumb flexion. In general, the superficial group arise from the common flexor origin (CFO) on the anterior aspect of the medial epicondyle of the humerus, as well as from adjacent bone and fascia.

Pronation

Pronator teres arises by two heads (the median nerve (12)) passing between, and therefore supplying them) from the CFO and the ulna. It passes to the convexity of the mid-shaft of the radius to roll it over the ulna in pronation. Pronator quadratus (13) is deeply and distally situated, passing between the anterior aspects of radius and ulna. It pronates as well as holding the radius and ulna in pronation. The anterior interosseous branch of the median nerve supplies them both, teres (C6,7) and quadratus (C8,T1).

Wrist flexion

Flexor carpi radialis (17) and flexor carpi ulnaris (18) arise from the CFO, but ulnaris also has a large ulnar head (the ulnar nerve (19) passes between the two heads of ulnaris and supplies them). Radialis passes posterior to the flexor retinaculum to attach to the bases of the second and third metacarpals, whereas ulnaris attaches via the pisiform to the hamate and

fifth metacarpal. Both flex the wrist but add radial or ulnar deviation, respectively. Palmaris longus (20) arises from the CFO and attaches to the flexor retinaculum and palmar aponeurosis to flex the wrist.

Flexor carpi ulnaris is supplied by the ulnar nerve (C8,T1), and the other two by the median nerve (C6,7,8). At the wrist the tendon of flexor carpi radialis has the median nerve medially and the radial artery (21) laterally.

Finger (digit) flexion

Flexor digitorum superficialis (22) arises from the CFO as well as the ulna, radius and overlying fascia. Flexor digitorum profundus (23) arises from the ulna and interosseous membrane. The tendons pass, in a synovial sheath, posterior to the flexor retinaculum (carpal tunnel) and into fibrous sheaths (24) anterior to the digits. Superficialis splits to attach to each side of the middle phalanges. Profundus passes through the split to attach to the base of the distal phalanges and is the only muscle to flex the distal interphalangeal joints. The muscles normally function together, to roll the fingers into flexion. But they must be tested individually when assessing injury. Holding three of a patient's fingers in extension prevents movement by profundus. Active flexion of the remaining finger is then only possible at the proximal interphalangeal joint and tests superficialis. Each finger must be assessed in turn. Active flexion of the distal interphalangeal joints individually tests profundus.

Superficialis is supplied by the median nerve, and profundus by the median for index and middle finger and the ulnar for ring and little fingers, i.e. the ulnar side of hand (C7,8,T1).

Thumb flexion

Flexor pollicis longus (26) from the radius and interosseous membrane passes posterior to the flexor retinaculum then, in fibrous and synovial sheaths, to insert onto the base of the distal phalanx. Assisted by flexor pollicis brevis (27), it flexes the thumb and is supplied by the median nerve (anterior interosseous branch) (C8,T1).

For the thumb and little finger the synovial sheaths in the digits are continuous with that in the carpal tunnel. This communication facilitates the spread of infection into the hand.

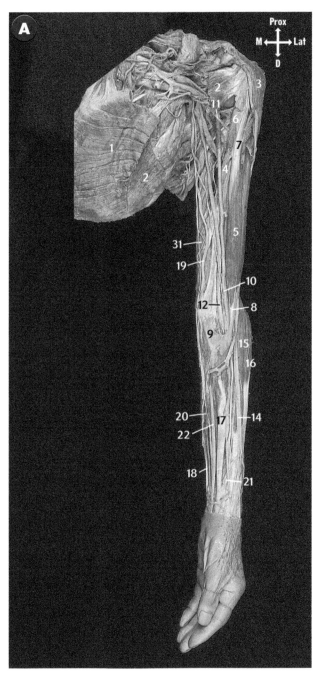

A　Muscles of the left upper limb (from the front)
B　Deep tendons, muscles of the left forearm and hand
(from the front)

1	Pectoralis major	10	Brachial artery
2	Pectoralis minor	11	Musculocutaneous nerve
3	Deltoid	12	Median nerve
4	Coracobrachialis	13	Pronator quadratus
5	Biceps	14	Cephalic vein
6	Short head of biceps, fused with coracobrachialis	15	Brachioradialis
7	Long head of biceps	16	Extensor carpi radialis longus
8	Tendon of biceps	17	Flexor carpi radialis
9	Bicipital aponeurosis	18	Flexor carpi ulnaris
		19	Ulnar nerve

20	Palmaris longus	28	Abductor digiti minimi
21	Radial artery	29	Flexor digiti minimi brevis
22	Flexor digitorum superficialis	30	Opponens digiti minimi
23	Tendons of flexor digitorum profundus in carpal tunnel	31	Triceps
24	Fibrous flexor sheath of index finger		
25	Abductor pollicis brevis		
26	Flexor pollicis longus		
27	Flexor pollicis brevis		

Location of numbers: 1A; 2A; 3A; 4A; 5A; 6A; 7A; 8A; 9A; 10A; 11A; 12A; 13B; 14A; 15A; 16A; 17AB; 18A; 19A; 20A; 21A; 22A; 23AB; 24B; 25B; 26B; 27B; 28B; 29B; 30B; 31A.

Upper limb: posterior muscle groups

Elbow extension

Triceps (1) arises by two heads from the humerus and one from the scapula (infraglenoid tubercle) to insert into the olecranon of the ulna. With a little help from anconeus, triceps extends the elbow. It is supplied by branches of the radial nerve (C6,7,8) that arise high in the axilla. The triceps reflex tests C7 and C8.

Muscles in the posterior aspect of the forearm are for: supination; wrist (carpal) extension, plus radial or ulnar deviation; finger (digit) extension; and thumb (pollicis) extension and abduction. Most arise from the common extensor origin (CEO) on the anterior aspect of humeral lateral epicondyle, and surrounding fascia. Functionally, brachioradialis (6) is an exception. It arises from the lateral supracondylar ridge of the humerus and passes to the lower end of the radius, just proximal to the styloid process. It is an elbow flexor, particularly when the forearm is in the midprone position. Nerve supply is from the radial (C5,6).

Supination

Supinator is a deeply situated muscle that arises from the CEO and the ulna. The posterior interosseous (deep) branch of the radial nerve passes between these two heads and supplies them. Supinator wraps around the posterior aspect of the radius to insert into its lateral surface. Its contraction 'unwinds' the pronated radius into supination. Like biceps, the other muscle that supinates, its segmental supply is C5,6.

Wrist extension

Power grip (e.g. holding a racket) is dependent on wrist extension, usually with radial deviation to counteract gravity. Therefore there are two extensors on the radial side and one on the ulnar. Extensor carpi radialis longus (7) arises from the CEO and the adjacent supracondylar ridge. It inserts into the second metacarpal. Extensor carpi radialis brevis (8) arises from the CEO to insert into the third metacarpal (the two extensor attachments mirror those of flexor carpi radialis). Extensor carpi ulnaris (9) arises from the CEO and ulna, to insert into the fifth metacarpal. All the muscles extend the wrist, with radial or ulnar deviation as the name implies. The radial nerve, or its posterior interosseous branch (C6,7,8) supplies these muscles.

Finger extension

Extensor digitorum (10) arises from the CEO and adjacent fascia, along with extensor digiti minimi (11), which runs parallel with it. Extensor indicis (12) arises from the ulna and interosseous membrane. The muscles form tendons that become the extensor expansions (13) inserting into all three phalanges of each finger to extend the metacarpophalangeal and interphalangeal joints. The index finger has two tendons, extensor digitorum and extensor indicis. The little finger also has two tendons, but these are derived from the divided tendon of extensor digiti minimi (14) with only a small contribution from extensor digitorum (15). Fibrous bands (intersections) (16) link the extensor tendons, making it difficult to extend individual fingers, except for the index (pointing) finger. The posterior interosseous nerve (C7,8) supplies all these muscles.

Thumb abduction and extension

These muscles originate deeply, and all have fibres arising from the interosseous membrane. Abductor pollicis longus (17) also arises from the ulna and radius; extensor pollicis longus (18) from the ulna; and extensor pollicis brevis (19) from the radius. The muscles become tendinous and pass to the thumb. Abductor longus runs with the extensor brevis but inserts into the base of the first metacarpal, while brevis inserts into the base of the proximal phalanx. Extensor longus glides around a tubercle on the posterior aspect of the radius, then inserts into the base of the distal phalanx of the thumb. The muscles abduct and extend the thumb, as implied by their names. The posterior interosseous nerve (C7,8) supplies them all.

The extensor retinaculum (20) arises from the radius and runs across the back of the wrist to the pisiform and hamate. All the above tendons run in synovial sheaths beneath the retinaculum. The sheaths commence proximal to the retinaculum but continue into the hand distally. **They may become inflamed due to excess activity (tenosynovitis).**

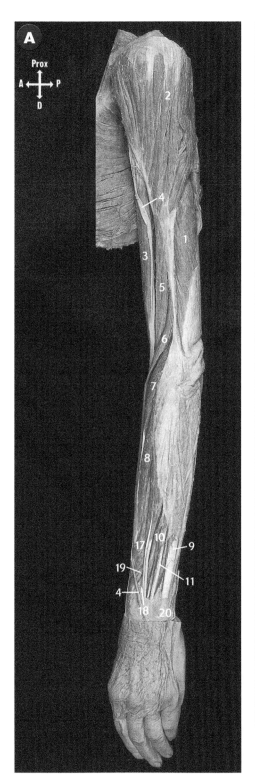

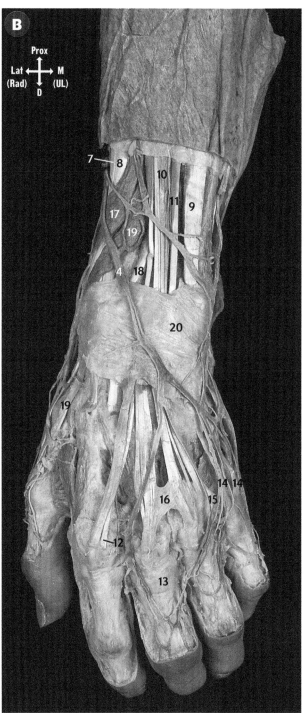

A Muscles of the left upper limb (from behind)
B Superficial dissection of the dorsum of the left hand
(from behind)

1	Triceps	**7**	Extensor carpi radialis longus	**13**	Extensor expansion	**16** Fibrous intersections between
2	Deltoid	**8**	Extensor carpi radialis brevis	**14**	Divided tendon of extensor digiti	extensor tendons
3	Biceps	**9**	Extensor carpi ulnaris		minimi	**17** Abductor pollicis longus
4	Cephalic vein	**10**	Extensor digitorum	**15**	Contribution of extensor	**18** Extensor pollicis longus
5	Coracobrachialis	**11**	Extensor digiti minimi		digitorum to extensor digiti	**19** Extensor pollicis brevis
6	Brachioradialis	**12**	Tendon of extensor indicis		minimi	**20** Extensor retinaculum

Location of numbers: **1**A; **2**A; **3**A; **4**AB; **5**A; **6**A; **7**AB; **8**AB; **9**AB; **10**AB; **11**AB; **12**B; **13**B; **14**B; **15**B; **16**B; **17**AB; **18**AB; **19**AB; **20**AB.

Superficial palm of hand, median nerve

The hand is for reaching out, touching, feeling (even identifying), manipulating and gripping. The skin is adherent to the underlying palmar aponeurosis (1), which receives palmaris longus (2) and passes from the flexor retinaculum (3) to the fibrous flexor sheaths of the fingers (4). The skin is highly sensitive. The palm may be 'cupped' for grip, aided by palmaris brevis (6) and the digits flex, extend, abduct and adduct. The thumb has the additional function of opposition.

Skin sensory supply is from the ulnar nerve (7) to the palmar and dorsal aspects of the medial (ulnar) side of the hand. It gives the dorsal and palmar digital branches (8) to both aspects of the medial (ulnar) one and a half digits, including the nail beds. The tip of the little finger is the ulnar nerve autonomous area. The remainder of the dorsum (except nail beds) is supplied by the radial nerve, the first dorsal web space being the autonomous area. The median nerve (11) supplies the palmar aspect of the lateral (radial) palm, and via its digital branches (12) the lateral three and half digits, including the nail beds. The tip of the index finger is the autonomous area.

The thenar and hypothenar eminences are created by the small muscles for the thumb and the equivalent ones (in brackets) for the little finger. These are: abductor pollicis brevis (14) (digiti minimi (15)); flexor pollicis brevis (16) (digiti minimi (17)); and more deeply opponens pollicis (opponens digiti minimi (18)). Objects may be held in the 'cup' of the palm, between the eminences.

The actions of the muscles (although limited for the little finger) are implied by the name. Hypothenar muscles (ulnar nerve) arise from the flexor retinaculum, pisiform and hamate. Thenar muscles (median nerve) arise from the flexor retinaculum, scaphoid and trapezium. Whatever the nerve supply, the root value is T1 (like all other small muscles in the hand). Thumb opposition is a uniquely human movement and dependent on the saddle-shaped first carpometacarpal joint. Opponens pollicis attaches to the length of the first metacarpal and swivels it to help carry the thumb into opposition. Flexor and abductor pollicis brevis attach to the proximal phalanx.

Median nerve

The median nerve (C5,6,7,8,T1) in the arm lies lateral to the brachial artery, but then crosses it to lie medial to the artery in the antecubital fossa. It then passes between the two heads of pronator teres to lie deep to flexor digitorum superficialis (19) in the forearm before passing through the carpal tunnel and into the hand.

The median nerve may be injured at the elbow. The thumb flexors are lost, as well as flexor digitorum superficialis to all fingers, and flexor profundus to the index and middle fingers. When asked to make a fist the patient can only flex the ring and little fingers, 'the hand of benediction'. Sensory loss may be variable due to nerve overlap, but there is always loss to the skin of the pulp over the distal phalanx of the index finger, i.e. the autonomous area of the median nerve. An extensive sensory loss to the hand following median nerve injury is particularly debilitating as patients injure (e.g. burn) themselves without realizing it, and manual dexterity is dependent on accurate sensation.

The long flexor tendons, in their common synovial sheath, pass into the palm behind the flexor retinaculum, a band of fibrous tissue from the pisiform and hook of hamate, across to the trapezium and scaphoid. Its proximal edge lies at the distal skin crease of the wrist. The ulnar nerve, and accompanying artery pass in a small canal of their own, anterior to the flexor retinaculum.

The median nerve runs with the tendons in the carpal tunnel (behind the retinaculum) where it may be compressed causing carpal tunnel syndrome. Signs and symptoms may include weakness and wasting of the thenar muscles with sensory disturbance over the radial three and half digits but not over the palm and thenar eminence. The latter skin areas are supplied by a superficial branch of the median nerve that arises proximal to, and passes into the palm, superficial to the flexor retinaculum.

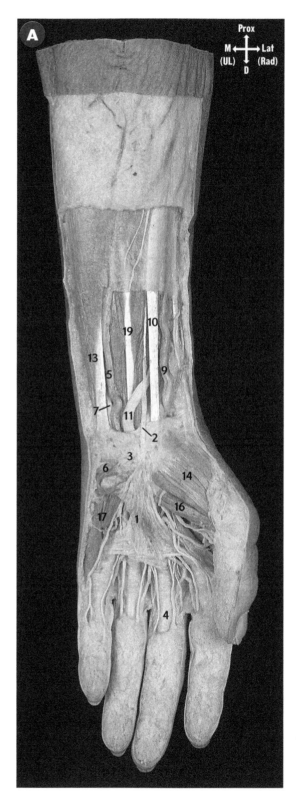

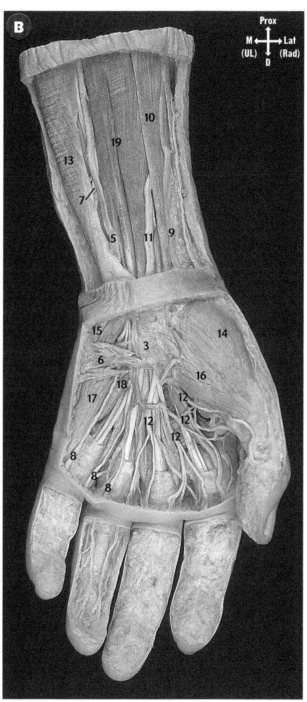

A Superficial structures of the left forearm and palm (from the front)

B Palm of the left hand, arteries and nerves (from the front)

1 Palmar aponeurosis	**6** Palmaris brevis	**11** Median nerve	**15** Abductor digiti minimi
2 Palmaris longus	**7** Ulnar nerve	**12** Digital branches of median	**16** Flexor pollicis brevis
3 Flexor retinaculum	**8** Digital branches of ulnar nerve	nerve	**17** Flexor digiti minimi brevis
4 Fibrous sheath of middle finger	**9** Radial artery	**13** Flexor carpi ulnaris	**18** Opponens digiti minimi
5 Ulnar artery	**10** Flexor carpi radialis	**14** Abductor pollicis brevis	**19** Flexor digitorum superficialis

Location of numbers: **1**A; **2**A; **3**AB; **4**A; **5**AB; **6**AB; **7**AB; **8**B; **9**AB; **10**AB; **11**AB; **12**B; **13**AB; **14**AB; **15**B; **16**AB; **17**AB; **18**B; **19**AB.

■ Deep palm, ulnar nerve, arteries

Muscles of the deep palm

Four lumbrical muscles (1) arise in the palm from the tendons of flexor digitorum profundus (2) and pass distally and posteriorly to attach to the radial aspect of the extensor tendon (expansion) of each finger. The medial (ulnar) two are bicipital and supplied by the ulnar nerve (5). The lateral (radial) two are unicipital and supplied by the median nerve (6).

Two sets of interosseous muscles arise between the metacarpal bones. Whatever the name or origin, like the lumbricals, they lie in the palm and pass anterior to the metacarpophalangeal joints. They attach to the proximal phalanges and the extensor expansions of the fingers. Palmar interossei adduct (palmar: PAD) the fingers toward the middle finger whereas dorsal interossei abduct (dorsal: DAB) the fingers away from that axis. The middle finger cannot adduct to itself, therefore does not have palmar interossei. As a result, there are three palmar interossei (8) passing one each to the side (closer to the middle finger) of the index, ring and little fingers. The middle finger can be abducted from its own axis therefore it has two dorsal interossei. So there are four dorsal interossei (9), one passing to each side of the middle finger, and one each to the side (away from the middle finger) of the index and ring fingers. The thumb and little finger do not need dorsal interossei as they have their own abductors (10,11). Similarly, the thumb does not need a palmar interosseous as it has its own adductor pollicis (12) passing from the carpal bones and third metacarpal to the base of the proximal phalanx. When the lumbricals and interossei function together, which is usual, they flex the metacarpophalangeal joints, because they pass anterior to them, and they extend the interphalangeal joints because they insert into the extensor expansions.

The deep branch of the ulnar nerve (13) supplies all the interossei and adductor pollicis. All small muscles of the hand are supplied by T1, via the ulnar nerve, except the lateral two lumbricals and the muscles of the thenar eminence (T1 via the median nerve).

Ulnar nerve

The ulnar nerve (C8,T1) lies medially in the arm, on triceps. It passes behind the medial humeral epicondyle and between the two heads of flexor carpi ulnaris before passing distally, medial to the ulnar artery (14), into the hand. The ulnar nerve may be injured as it passes posterior to the medial epicondyle, or at the wrist where it is superficial to the flexor retinaculum in the canal of Guyon. Injury to the ulnar causes loss of all interossei and the two medial lumbricals, as well as adductor pollicis. Therefore, the two medial fingers form an 'ulnar claw': extended at the metacarpophalangeal joints and flexed at the interphalangeal joints as a result of loss of interphalangeal extension and metacarpophalangeal flexion (the combined actions of the lumbricals and interossei). This is less marked if the injury is at the elbow as flexor digitorum profundus is also lost. The fingers cannot be abducted from the axis of the middle finger (dorsal interossei) or adducted toward it (palmar interossei). Thumb adduction is lost and if patients are asked to hold a sheet of paper by adducting the thumb to the palm, they will use the thumb flexors, which are supplied by the median nerve (Froment's sign).

Palmar arteries

The ulnar and radial arteries (15) pass into the palm. The ulnar runs anteriorly, but the radial courses posteriorly before it passes between the first two metacarpals to enter the palm in a deep position. Branches of the arteries anastomose to form superficial and deep palmar arches (16). The latter lies deep to the long tendons, whereas the former is anterior. The superficial arch lies opposite the cleft of the outstretched thumb, the deep arch about one fingerbreadth proximally.

The arches give metacarpal arteries (17) that divide to give both dorsal and palmar digital arteries (18) to each side of the digit. Digital nerves (19,20) accompany these. Injury to the anastomotic palmar arches may cause profuse bleeding. The digital nerves may be anaesthetized (ring block) to carry out minor operations on the digits.

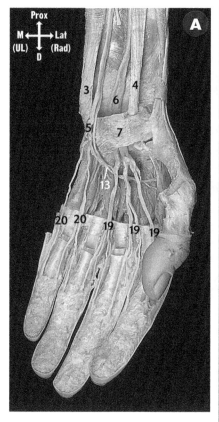

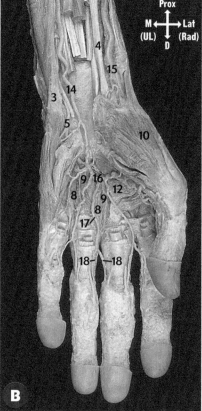

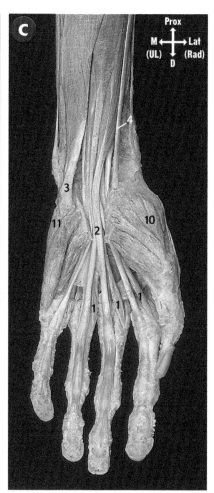

A Deep dissection of left palm, nerve supply (from the front)
B Deep dissection of left palm, arterial supply (from the front)
C Deep dissection of left palm, muscles and tendons (from the front)

1	Lumbrical muscles	**6**	Median nerve
2	Tendons of flexor digitorum	**7**	Flexor retinaculum
	profundus in carpal tunnel	**8**	Palmar interossei
3	Flexor carpi ulnaris	**9**	Dorsal interossei
4	Flexor carpi radialis	**10**	Abductor pollicis brevis
5	Ulnar nerve	**11**	Abductor digiti minimi

12	Adductor pollicis	**18**	Palmar digital artery
13	Deep branch of ulnar nerve	**19**	Digital branches of median
14	Ulnar artery		nerve
15	Radial artery	**20**	Digital branches of ulnar nerve
16	Deep palmar arch		
17	Metacarpal artery		

Location of numbers: **1**C; **2**C; **3**ABC; **4**ABC; **5**AB; **6**A; **7**A; **8**B; **9**B; **10**BC; **11**C; **12**B; **13**A; **14**B; **15**B; **16**B; **17**B; **18**B; **19**A; **20**A.

Axillary artery, brachial plexus, radial nerve

Axillary artery

The **axillary artery with vein (1,2)** medially, is the continuation of the subclavian as it passes over the first rib. It becomes the **brachial artery (3)** at the inferior edge of **teres major (4)**. The axillary artery supplies branches to the muscles on the chest wall, the arm, and those that bound the **axilla (5–11)**. Its branches provide important contributions to anastomoses around the scapula and the elbow. In the female its **lateral thoracic branch (12)** is an important blood supply to the breast.

Brachial plexus

The plexus is formed by the ventral rami of spinal nerves C5–8 and T1. These are the roots of the brachial plexus that supplies the upper limb. C5–8 emerge into the neck between scalenus anterior and medius. T1 emerges inferior to the neck of the first rib, but joins the plexus above the apex of the lung.

C5 and C6 form the upper trunk, C7 continues as the middle trunk, while C8 and T1 form the lower trunk. The trunks pass laterally and lie around the subclavian artery while passing over the first rib to enter the axilla, between the clavicle and the scapula. Behind the clavicle, each trunk splits into anterior and posterior divisions. These recombine to form the **posterior (13)**, **lateral (14)** and **medial (15)** cords around the axillary artery. The upper roots (C5–7) tend to stay lateral, the lower roots (C8,T1) tend to stay medial. All roots contribute to the posterior cord, and therefore also to the radial nerve. The median nerve is formed from both lateral and medial cords, therefore also contains all roots. Proximal muscles tend to be supplied by nerve roots that emerge from higher segments of the spinal cord. Distal muscles are supplied by nerves arising from the lower segments. The five main branches of the brachial plexus are **median (16)**, **ulnar (17)**, **radial (18)**, **axillary (19)** and **musculocutaneous (20)** nerves.

Branches from both lateral and medial cords supply the pectoral muscles. After supplying the pectorals and contributing to the median nerve, the lateral cord becomes the musculocutaneous nerve. Subscapularis, teres major and latissimus dorsi are supplied by the posterior cord, which also gives the axillary nerve to deltoid and teres minor before continuing as the radial nerve. The medial cord contributes to the median nerve, and also gives cutaneous nerves to the medial arm and forearm before continuing as the ulnar nerve.

Upper trunk injury removes C5 and C6, which supply the shoulder abductors and external rotators, and the elbow flexors and supinators. Consequently, the upper limb lies at the side adducted and internally rotated. The elbow is extended and pronated. The fingers may flex slightly and the condition, Erb's palsy, is often called 'waiter's tip' palsy. Lower trunk injury (Klumpke's paralysis) removes C8 and T1, therefore all the thenar and hypothenar muscles are affected, along with the lumbricals and interossei. The hand is flattened and the fingers clawed.

Radial nerve

The radial nerve (C5–8,T1) as well as sending cutaneous branches to the posterior aspects of arm and forearm, supplies triceps, and its posterior interosseous branch supplies the wrist, finger and thumb extensors. The radial nerve may be injured as it winds posteriorly around the midshaft of the humerus. If so, triceps will be spared as the nerve supply arises in the axilla, but wrist and finger extension will be lost. The main disability is the loss of power grip, as that depends on wrist extension. There will be sensory loss over the first dorsal web space, the autonomous area of the radial nerve.

In the antecubital region the radial nerve lies deep to brachioradialis. After giving the posterior interosseous branch it continues into the forearm lying lateral to the radial artery, to supply the skin of the dorsum of the hand and radial three and a half digits (but not the nail beds). The posterior interosseous passes between the two heads of supinator (therefore supplies it) and continues to supply all the muscles in the extensor aspect of the forearm. It lies close to the radius and may be injured in fractures of that bone or during surgical plating of the fracture.

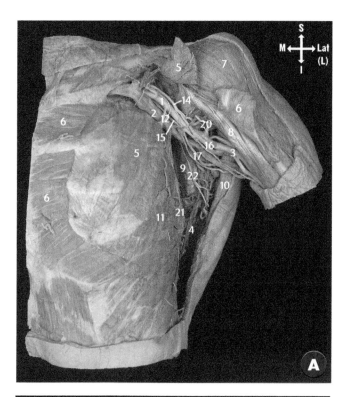

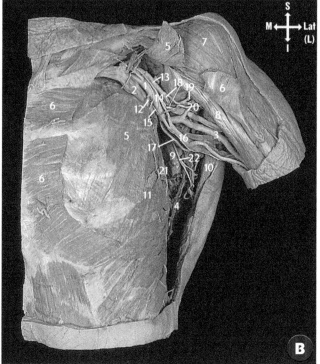

A Left axilla and brachial plexus (from the left and front)
B Left axilla and brachial plexus with displacement of
   nerves (from the left and front)

1	Axillary artery	7	Deltoid	13	Posterior cord	19	Axillary nerve
2	Axillary vein	8	Short head of biceps	14	Lateral cord	20	Musculocutaneous nerve
3	Brachial artery	9	Subscapularis	15	Medial cord	21	Long thoracic nerve
4	Teres major	10	Latissimus dorsi	16	Median nerve	22	Thoracodorsal nerve
5	Pectoralis minor	11	Serratus anterior	17	Ulnar nerve		
6	Pectoralis major	12	Lateral thoracic artery	18	Radial nerve		

Location of numbers: **1**AB; **2**AB; **3**AB; **4**AB; **5**AB; **6**AB; **7**AB; **8**AB; **9**AB; **10**AB; **11**AB; **12**AB; **13**B; **14**AB; **15**AB; **16**AB; **17**AB; **18**B; **19**B; **20**AB; **21**AB; **22**AB.

Part IX

The Lower Limb

Lower limb: fascia, superficial veins, sural nerve, lymph nodes

Deep fascia

The deep fascia (1) is like a stocking encompassing the whole lower limb. In the thigh it is named fascia lata, which attaches to the inguinal ligament (2) and also to the bony prominences: iliac crest, ischium, pubic arch, femoral condyles. The fascia lata is continuous with the deep fascia of the leg, attaching to the tibial condyles, head of fibula and subcutaneous border of the tibia (3). At the ankle it is specialized to form flexor, extensor and fibular (peroneal) retinacula (4), before continuing with the fascia of the foot. In the thigh fascia lata is thinner medially and has an opening (cribriform fascia) to transmit the great saphenous vein (5). Laterally it is thickened to form the iliotibial tract (8), which runs from the ilium to the upper anterior part of the lateral tibial condyle. It receives two muscles and is an important stabilizer of both hip and knee joints, therefore of the lower limb.

Intermuscular septa pass from the deep fascia to lie between muscles and provide muscle origin as well as definite compartments. In the thigh septa separate the quadriceps and adductor muscles from the hamstrings. Sartorius (10) has a layer of fascia separating it from the underlying muscles and forming the subsartorial canal, which transmits the femoral vessels on their way to pierce adductor magnus and continue as popliteal vessels. In the leg, particularly the calf, the fascial compartmentalization ensures that as muscles contract the deep veins are compressed, aiding venous return to the heart (the muscle pump). But muscle damage or bone fracture may cause swelling that becomes restricted within the compartment. In turn the raised pressure will constrict and obstruct neurovascular supply. Such compartment syndrome often must be released surgically by cutting the fascia before muscle ischaemia and necrosis occur.

Superficial veins of the lower limb

The veins are divided into superficial and deep groups. The superficial veins are variable but do consistently show the great (long) and small (short) saphenous veins. All veins have valves and flow is from superficial, via perforators to the deep system, which parallels the arteries, and then proximally. The superficial veins also freely communicate with each other.

The great saphenous vein starts on the dorsum of the foot. It passes 2 cm anterior to the medial malleolus (11) where it is constant. It may be approached, by cutting down through the skin, for emergency venous access. The saphenous nerve, lying alongside, may be severed causing sensory deficit on the medial border of the foot. The vein ascends up the medial leg to lie immediately posterior to the medial femoral condyle (one hand-breadth behind the patella). It then passes up the medial thigh and through the cribriform fascia, 2.5 cm below and lateral to the pubic tubercle, to enter the femoral vein (12). It receives a number of tributaries just before passing through the fascia. These must be identified during varicose vein surgery.

The great saphenous has perforators, with valves, around the ankle and knee. Should the valves become incompetent blood may flow from deep to superficial and the superficial veins become tortuous and dilated (varicose veins). This slows venous return, leading ultimately to skin changes around the ankle (lipodermatosclerosis), which may ulcerate following injury. Varicose veins may bleed profusely if injured.

The small saphenous vein (13) passes behind the lateral malleolus (14) and ascends up the posterior aspect of the calf to enter the popliteal vein (15) behind the knee. The sural nerve (16) is derived from both the tibial (17) and common fibular (18) nerves. It lies with the small saphenous vein and supplies the skin of the posterior calf and lateral border of the foot. The sural may be harvested for nerve grafting.

Lymph nodes

These are found in the popliteal fossa and inguinal region. The superficial inguinal are in two groups that form a 'T' at the upper end of the great saphenous vein, and parallel with, but just inferior to the inguinal ligament. They drain to the deep inguinal nodes just medial to the femoral vein, and through the femoral canal to the iliac nodes.

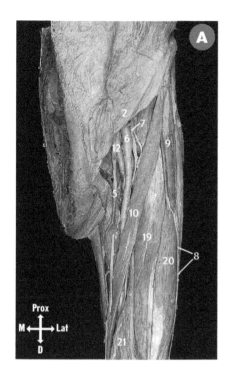

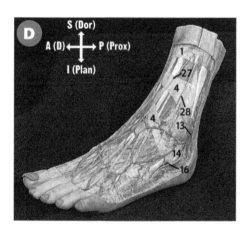

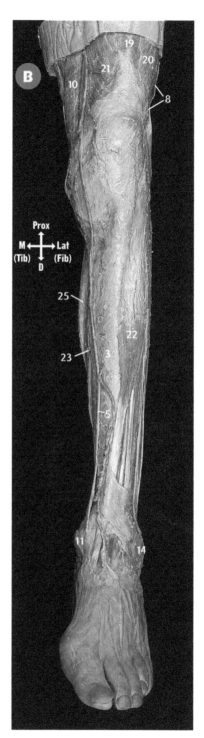

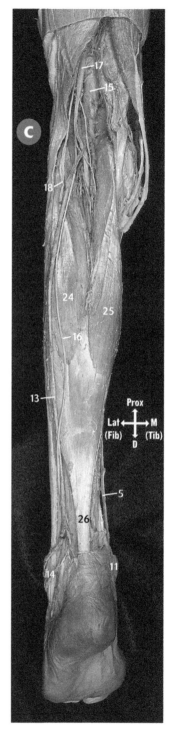

A **Left thigh (from the front)**
B **Left lower limb superficial structures (from the front)**
C **Left lower limb superficial structures (from behind)**
D **Left foot (from the front and left)**

1	Deep fascia of the leg	9	Tensor fasciae latae	18	Common fibular (peroneal) nerve	26	Calcaneal tendon (Achilles tendon)
2	External oblique aponeurosis becoming the inguinal ligament	10	Sartorius	19	Rectus femoris	27	Medial branch of superficial fibular (peroneal) nerve
3	Shaft of tibia	11	Medial malleolus	20	Vastus lateralis	28	Lateral branch of superficial fibular (peroneal) nerve
4	Retinacula	12	Femoral vein	21	Vastus medialis		
5	Great saphenous vein	13	Small saphenous vein	22	Tibialis anterior		
6	Femoral artery	14	Lateral malleolus	23	Soleus		
7	Femoral nerve	15	Popliteal vein	24	Lateral head of gastrocnemius		
8	Cut edge of iliotibial tract	16	Sural nerve	25	Medial head of gastrocnemius		
		17	Tibial nerve				

Location of numbers: **1**D; **2**A; **3**B; **4**D; **5**ABC; **6**A; **7**A; **8**AB; **9**A; **10**AB; **11**BC; **12**A; **13**C; **14**BCD; **15**C; **16**CD; **17**C; **18**C; **19**AB; **20**AB; **21**AB; **22**B; **23**B; **24**C; **25**BC; **26**C; **27**D; **28**D.

Hip joint, prevention of pelvic tilt

Hip joint

As the pelvic girdle is barely flexible, movement of the lower limb is largely at the hip joint, which also transmits the body weight. When compared with the shoulder, the synovial ball and socket hip has increased stability but reduced mobility. The head of the femur (1) lies within the deep socket of the acetabulum (2); itself deepened by the fibrocartilage labrum (3). The femoral head is offset from the femoral shaft (4) by the femoral neck (5), which means all hip movements become rotation of the head within the acetabulum.

The fibrous capsule (6) arises from the acetabular margins and the labrum. It passes laterally to enclose the head and much of the neck of the femur. Anteriorly it attaches to the intertrochanteric line but posteriorly falls short of the intertrochanteric crest to leave space for the insertion of the lateral rotator muscles onto the femoral neck and the medial aspect of the greater trochanter (7). As the capsule attaches to the femoral neck fibres pass medially up the neck toward the head. These retinacular fibres carry the blood supply to the femoral head.

Ligaments arising from the three elements of the hip bone strengthen the capsule. The ilio-, pubo- and ischiofemoral ligaments arise adjacent to the acetabulum and pass, as part of the capsule, to insert into the femoral neck and intertrochanteric line. As humans have adapted to stand erect the hip joint is already extended, and any further extension is limited. The ligaments tend to spiral around the joint and are particularly supportive in this upright position. The ligament of the head of the femur (8) passes from the acetabulum to the femoral head and may carry some blood supply, particularly in the young.

Hip movements

Hip flexion. Iliopsoas (9,10,11) arises from the lumbar vertebrae and intervening discs, and from the inner aspect of the ilium, to attach to the lesser trochanter. Psoas is supplied segmentally mainly by L1 and L2, and iliacus by L2 and L3 via the femoral nerve.

Hip adduction. Pectineus (12), adductor longus (13) and brevis (14), and magnus arise from the pubis and ischium, and attach to the femur. Gracilis (15), also from the pubis, passes to the tibia and has additional functions of knee flexion and internal rotation of the tibia. The small, tendinous origin of adductor longus is the site of 'groin strain'.

The obturator nerve (L2–4 anterior divisions) emerges from the medial side of psoas major in the pelvis. It passes on the lateral pelvic wall, then through the obturator foramen and into the medial thigh. It splits into two branches, one on either side of adductor brevis and supplies all the adductors (except pectineus, which is femoral) and the skin of the medial thigh. If it is injured some adduction remains via the sciatic supply to magnus. Branches of the femoral and obturator nerves supply both the hip and knee therefore the two joints may refer pain to each other.

Prevention of pelvic tilt

During walking, or standing on one leg gravity makes the body topple to the unsupported side. The adductors act synergistically with the hip abductors (18,19) and the iliotibial tract to support the weight of the body and hold the pelvis level. The neck of the femur gives mechanical advantage to the abductors. Shortening of the neck (congenital dislocation of the hip, prosthetic hip) will weaken the supportive effect of the abductors and the pelvis will dip to the opposite side when walking (Trendelenburg gait).

Fractures of the neck of the femur, within the capsule, usually tear the retinacular fibres, cutting off the blood supply to the femoral head and causing avascular necrosis. Iliopsoas pulls the lower limb upward and externally rotates it, as the axis of movement following the fracture is through the femoral shaft. The limb appears shortened and the foot laterally rotated. Severe trauma may cause a posterior dislocation of the hip that may fracture a small piece of bone from the acetabulum. That bony fragment may damage the sciatic nerve, which lies immediately behind the joint. A central dislocation occurs when severe trauma pushes the femoral head through the acetabulum.

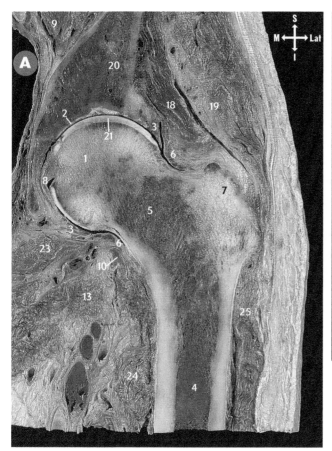

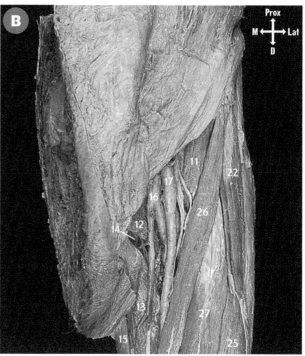

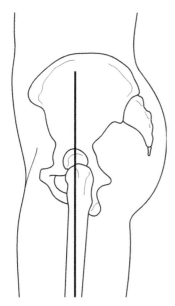

A   Coronal section through the left hip joint (from the front)
B   Left thigh (from the front)

Line diagram adapted from Ellis H, Logan BM, Dixon AK (2001) *Human Sectional Anatomy*. London: Arnold.

1 Head of femur	**8** Ligament of the head of femur	**14** Adductor brevis	**21** Articular cartilage
2 Rim of acetabulum	(ligamentum teres)	**15** Gracilis	**22** Tensor fasciae latae
3 Acetabular labrum	**9** Psoas major	**16** Femoral vein	**23** Obturator externus
4 Shaft of femur	**10** Iliopsoas tendon	**17** Femoral artery	**24** Vastus medialis
5 Neck of femur	**11** Iliacus	**18** Gluteus minimus	**25** Vastus lateralis
6 Capsule of hip joint	**12** Pectineus	**19** Gluteus medius	**26** Sartorius
7 Greater trochanter	**13** Adductor longus	**20** Ilium	**27** Rectus femoris

Location of numbers: **1**A; **2**A; **3**A; **4**A; **5**A; **6**A; **7**A; **8**A; **9**A; **10**A; **11**B; **12**B; **13**AB; **14**B; **15**B; **16**B; **17**B; **18**A; **19**A; **20**A; **21**A; **22**B; **23**A; **24**A; **25**AB; **26**B; **27**B.

Knee joint

The knee is a synovial, modified hinge joint between the femur (1) and the tibia (2). Movements are essentially flexion and extension, but rotation is possible when the knee is flexed. The patella (3) is a sesamoid bone in the tendon of quadriceps (4,5), and it articulates with the femur. The lateral articular surface of the patella is larger than the medial. The femoral condyles (6) are rounded. Anteriorly the lateral condyle is more prominent than the medial to counteract the natural tendency for quadriceps to draw the patella in a lateral direction during knee extension. The upper end of the tibia (7) is a flat plateau with an intercondylar eminence.

The fibrous capsule attaches to the articular margins of the femur and tibia. It is created from ligaments, from extensions of the tendons around the joint, and by the patella. Extensions of the quadriceps, the patellar retinacula, pass between the patella and the tibia. Laterally, fibres from the iliotibial tract similarly strengthen the capsule. Posteromedially, it is strengthened by the oblique popliteal ligament and semimembranosus (8), and posterolaterally, the capsule is strengthened by the arcuate popliteal ligament that arises from the head of the fibula. These tendinous extensions ensure tension of the capsule. Many of the tendons around the joint have bursae between them, the capsule and its ligaments, or other tendons. There are subcutaneous bursae (9) over the patella and over the ligamentum patella, as well as a deep bursa between the tibia and the ligamentum patella. All the bursae may become inflamed, swollen and tender. The joint extends upward behind quadriceps as the suprapatellar bursa (11).

Ligaments

The knee, like all hinge joints, is supported by collateral ligaments. The medial collateral is a band that is part of the capsule and runs from the medial femoral epicondyle to the tibia. The lateral collateral is cord-like and separate from the capsule. It passes from the lateral femoral epicondyle to the fibula (splitting the tendon of biceps femoris).

The cruciate ligaments are within the knee joint, but invaginated into the synovium from behind, therefore outside the synovial sheath. The anterior cruciate (12) arises from the anterior aspect of the tibial intercondylar area and passes to the internal aspect of the lateral femoral condyle. The posterior cruciate (13) arises from the posterior tibial intercondylar area and passes to the inner aspect of the medial femoral condyle. The two ligaments cross each other and are taut in extension. The anterior prevents excessive forward movement of the tibia; the posterior prevents excessive posterior movement. Lateral blows (car bumper) to the extended knee tend to damage the anterior cruciate ligament, the medial collateral ligament and with it the medial meniscus. Injuries to the posterior cruciate ligament leave a patient with difficulty walking downstairs as the femur may slide forward on the tibia.

The fibrocartilage menisci are between the femur and tibia, making the joint surfaces more congruent and acting as shock absorbers. They are crescentic-shaped wedges that attach to the tibial intercondylar area by their 'horns' but peripherally attach to the joint capsule. They move during flexion and extension of the knee, but the medial meniscus (14,15) is restricted as it is, via its capsular attachment, also attached to the medial collateral ligament, which is part of the capsule. The menisci, particularly the medial, may be injured when the femur is traumatically forced to rotate on the femur with the knee extended.

As the knee moves normally into full extension, the femur rotates medially around the axis of the cruciate (particularly anterior) ligaments. The knee is then 'close-packed' so that the lower limb becomes a supportive strut with only minimal continued use of quadriceps and of the iliotibial tract.

Popliteus (23) must laterally rotate the femur at the start of knee flexion. It arises from the posterior aspect of the tibia. Its tendon passes through the joint capsule, sends a slip to the lateral meniscus (that moves it), before inserting onto the lateral femoral condyle, below the epicondyle. Nerve supply is via the tibial nerve (24) (L4,5,S1).

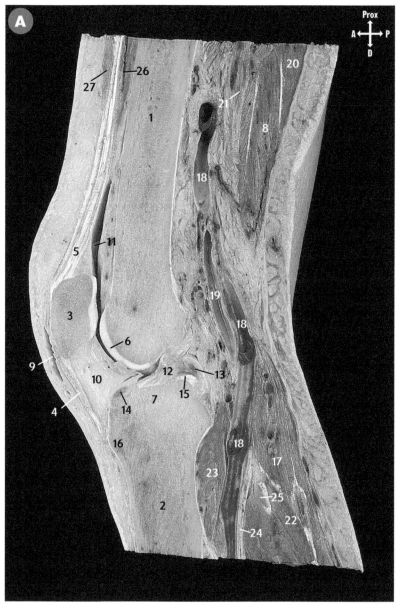

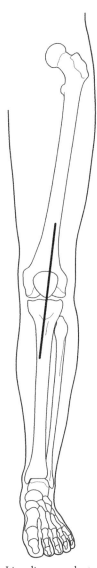

Line diagram adapted from Ellis H, Logan BM, Dixon AK (2001) *Human Sectional Anatomy*. London: Arnold.

A Sagittal section through the left knee from the left

1	Shaft of femur	7	Proximal end of tibia (tibial plateau)	14	Anterior horn of medial meniscus	21	Sciatic nerve
2	Shaft of tibia	8	Semimembranosus	15	Posterior horn of medial meniscus	22	Soleus
3	Patella	9	Prepatellar bursa			23	Popliteus
4	Patellar ligament (ligamentum patellae)	10	Infrapatellar pad of fat extending into infrapatellar fold	16	Tibial tuberosity	24	Tibial nerve
5	Tendon of quadriceps femoris	11	Suprapatellar bursa	17	Gastrocnemius	25	Tendon of plantaris
6	Articular cartilage on medial femoral condyle	12	Anterior cruciate ligament	18	Popliteal vein	26	Vastus intermedius
		13	Posterior cruciate ligament	19	Popliteal artery	27	Rectus femoris
				20	Semitendinosus		

Tibiofibular, ankle and tarsal joints, arches of foot

Tibiofibular joints

The tibia (1) and fibula (2) are held together by the interosseous membrane. Superiorly there is a synovial joint between the tibia and the head of the fibula. Inferiorly there is a fibrous joint, supported by further ligaments situated anteriorly and posteriorly.

Ankle joint

At their lower ends, the tibia and fibula clasp the talus (3) to form the ankle joint (4). The tibia is the medial-malleolus (5), while the arrow-shaped inferior end of the fibula is the lateral malleolus (6). The talus (and therefore the foot) moves only in dorsiflexion (extension) and plantarflexion (flexion) between the malleoli. The ankle joint capsule attaches to the articular margins. As expected in a hinge joint, it is lax anteriorly and posteriorly, but strengthened at the sides by collateral ligaments.

The strong medial collateral (deltoid) ligament (7) is like a triangle with its apex at the medial malleolus and the base formed by its attachment to the navicular (8), spring ligament, sustentaculum tali (calcaneus) and talus. The lateral ligament is in three separate bands. Splaying from the lateral malleolus are: anterior talofibular (9) to the neck of the talus; calcaneofibular to the calcaneus (a band separate from the capsule); the posterior talofibular passing backward to the lateral tubercle on the posterior aspect of the talus.

 Injury to the ankle ligaments, particularly on the lateral aspect is common. The bruising, swelling and tenderness may vary depending on which band has been injured. Fractures around the ankle may affect the joint surface, possibly causing the early onset of arthritis, with consequent painful limitation to walking and running. Severe injury may also disrupt the inferior tibiofibular joint. The trochlear surface of the talus is wider anteriorly and if the ankle is immobilized in plaster the foot must be dorsiflexed so that the broader part of the talus is in the 'socket' between the tibia and fibula. The posterior tibial neurovascular bundle lies behind and below the medial malleolus and may be at risk in fractures and dislocation of the ankle.

Tarsal joints

The foot has a series of joints between all the tarsal bones. These may be simplified and collectively referred to as the subtarsal joint, which includes: talus to calcaneus and navicular; calcaneus to cuboid (10,11) (sometimes called midtarsal). These joints are synovial, have fibrous capsules and are supported by ligaments. They allow for inversion and eversion of the foot.

Arches of the foot

The arches are formed naturally as the bones of the foot articulate with each other. Each foot has a longitudinal arch, described as having medial and lateral components. The medial arch of calcaneus (12), talus, navicular, cuneiforms (13) and the three medial metatarsals (14) is highly arched before reaching the ground again at the metatarsal heads and phalanges (15,16). The head of the talus (19) is the highest point, or keystone of the arch. The lateral arch of calcaneus and cuboid to the lateral two metatarsals and phalanges is much lower. Each foot forms half of a transverse arch, which is complete when the feet are placed together.

As well as the ligaments and small muscles, the long tendons within the sole also support the arches. Tibialis anterior and posterior hold up the medial arch, which is also supported by the tendon of flexor hallucis longus (20) and the plantar aponeurosis (21). Fibularis (peroneus) longus and brevis support the lateral longitudinal arch, but the tendon of longus passes in a groove beneath the cuboid to insert into the medial cuneiform and first metatarsal, therefore also maintaining the transverse arch.

The arches act as shock absorbers but are also important in the propulsive phases of walking and running, where traction on the plantar aponeurosis makes them become higher.

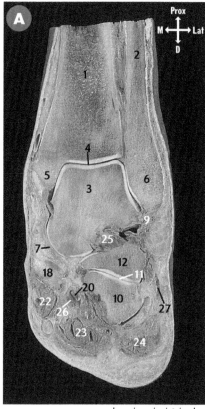

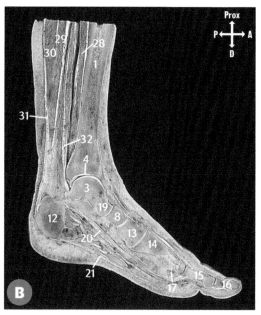

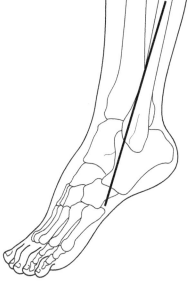

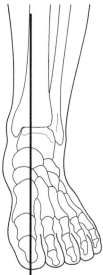

A Coronal section through the left ankle joint and foot
(from the front) with the foot in plantarflexion

B Sagittal section through the left foot (from the right)

Line diagrams adapted from Ellis H, Logan BM, Dixon AK (2001)
Human Sectional Anatomy. London: Arnold.

1	Tibia	10	Cuboid
2	Fibula	11	Calcaneocuboid joint
3	Talus	12	Calcaneus
4	Ankle joint	13	Medial cuneiform
5	Medial malleolus	14	First metatarsal bone
6	Lateral malleolus	15	Proximal phalanx of hallux
7	Medial collateral (deltoid) ligament	16	Distal phalanx of hallux
8	Navicular	17	Sesamoid bone
9	Anterior talofibular (lateral collateral) ligament of ankle	18	Tendon of tibialis posterior
		19	Head of talus

20	Tendon of flexor hallucis longus	27	Tendon of fibularis (peroneus) brevis
21	Plantar aponeurosis	28	Flexor digitorum longus
22	Abductor hallucis	29	Soleus
23	Flexor digitorum brevis	30	Gastrocnemius
24	Abductor digiti minimi	31	Calcaneal (Achilles) tendon
25	Talocalcaneal interosseous ligament	32	Flexor hallucis longus
26	Tendon of flexor digitorum longus		

Location of numbers: 1AB; 2A; 3AB; 4AB; 5A; 6A; 7A; 8B; 9A; 10A; 11A; 12AB; 13B; 14B; 15B; 16B; 17B; 18A; 19B; 20AB; 21B; 22A; 23A; 24A; 25A; 26A; 27A; 28B; 29B; 30B; 31B; 32B.

Sole of foot: plantar aponeurosis, muscle layers, neurovascular supply

Plantar aponeurosis

Although the functions of the palm and sole are different, the topography is similar. The thick plantar skin attaches to the underlying plantar aponeurosis (1), which passes forward from the tuberosity on the posterior aspect of the inferior surface of the calcaneus to attach to the fibrous flexor sheaths of each toe. The aponeurosis sends septa into the foot. These create compartments and give origin to some of the small muscles of the sole. The most important function of the plantar aponeurosis is maintenance of the longitudinal arch. In walking, the toes are forced into dorsiflexion, pulling on the aponeurosis, and in turn pulling on the calcaneus to heighten the arch.

Muscle layers

The muscles in the sole move the toes and support the arches. They are arranged in layers, like the palm. The superficial layer is formed by abductors hallucis (2) and digiti minimi (3), which have minimal actions suggested by their names, and lie on either side of flexor digitorum brevis (4) (equivalent to flexor digitorum superficialis (forearm)). It arises from the calcaneus and passes forward as the four tendons for the lateral toes. These tendons run into fibrous sheaths, split to allow the passage of flexor digitorum longus and insert into the sides of the middle phalanges.

The second layer contains flexor digitorum longus (7) that gives origin to the lumbricals (8), and receives flexor accessorius (9), which arises from the calcaneus and inserts into the tendons of longus to straighten their oblique pull. The tendon of flexor hallucis longus (10) passes into the sole, immediately inferior to the sustentaculum tali and the spring (plantar calcaneonavicular) ligament. It lies superior to the tendons of flexor digitorum longus before running forward to enter the fibrous flexor sheath of the hallux and insert into the base of the distal phalanx. It flexes the hallux and gives powerful propulsion in walking.

The third layer contains flexor hallucis brevis (12) and flexor digiti minimi brevis (13), which lie on either side of adductor hallucis. Both arise from the tarsal bones and ligaments, insert into the proximal phalanges and carry out the actions indicated by their names. Flexor hallucis brevis attaches to both sides of the phalanx and the tendons may contain sesamoids.

The fourth, and deepest, layer contains the plantar and dorsal interossei, which adduct and abduct around the axis of the second toe.

Neurovascular supply

The posterior tibial neurovascular bundle passes into the sole above flexor digitorum brevis. The tibial nerve (14) divides into medial (15) and lateral (16) plantar nerves, equivalent to the median and ulnar nerves.

The medial plantar nerve supplies the small muscles for the big toe (except the adductor) and flexor digitorum brevis (median nerve supplies superficialis in the forearm and the thenar muscles). It also supplies only the first lumbrical, as the axis for the foot is the second toe rather than the middle one. The lateral plantar supplies all the other muscles, including flexor accessorius (which does not have an equivalent in the hand), adductor hallucis, all the interossei and the lateral three lumbricals. Although rare, injury to the lateral plantar nerve may cause clawing of the foot.

Much of the skin on the medial sole and medial three and half toes (including nail beds), is supplied by the medial plantar nerve, and on the lateral aspect and lateral one and half toes (and nail beds) by the lateral plantar. Skin on the medial border of the foot is supplied by the saphenous nerve, whereas the sural nerve supplies the lateral border and heel. Whatever the nerve supply, the muscles of the sole are supplied by S1,2,3 and the dermatomes are L4,5 and S1 from medial to lateral.

The posterior tibial artery (17) divides into medial (smaller) and lateral plantar (larger) branches. They pass above flexor digitorum brevis to supply the foot and toes. The lateral plantar forms a plantar arcade with a branch coming between the metatarsals from the dorsalis pedis. Metatarsal branches from the arcade send plantar digital arteries to the toes. An arcade on the dorsum, from the anterior tibial artery, sends dorsal metatarsal and dorsal digital arteries.

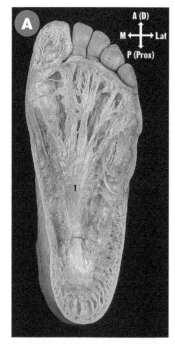

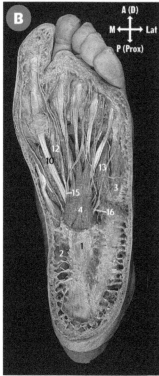

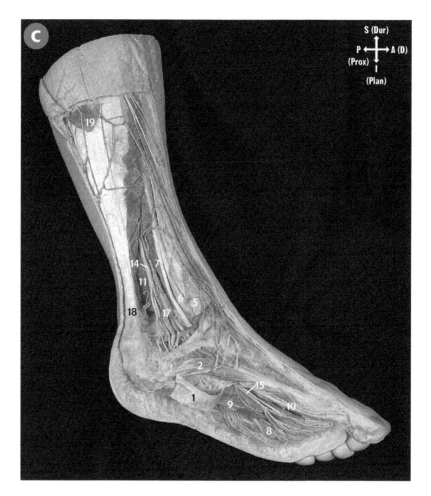

A Sole of left foot superficial from below
B Sole of left foot first and second layer from below
C Left leg and sole of foot second layer from the right and below

1	Plantar aponeurosis	6	Tibialis posterior	10	Tendon of flexor hallucis longus	15	Medial plantar nerve
2	Abductor hallucis	7	Flexor digitorum longus	11	Flexor hallucis longus	16	Lateral plantar nerve
3	Abductor digiti minimi	8	Lumbrical	12	Flexor hallucis brevis	17	Posterior tibial artery and veins
4	Flexor digitorum brevis	9	Quadratus plantae (flexor accessorius)	13	Flexor digiti minimi brevis	18	Calcaneal (Achilles) tendon
5	Medial malleolus of tibia			14	Tibial nerve	19	Gastrocnemius

Location of numbers: 1ABC; 2BC; 3B; 4B; 5C; 6C; 7C; 8C; 9C; 10BC; 11C; 12B; 13B; 14C; 15BC; 16B; 17C; 18C; 19C.

Lower limb: anterior muscle groups

Knee extension

Quadriceps: vastus medialis (1), lateralis (2) and intermedius arise from the femur; rectus femoris (3) arises from the ilium and overlies intermedius. They insert via the patella (4), into the tibial tuberosity (5) to extend the knee. Rectus femoris also flexes the hip (the kicking muscle). The lower fibres of medialis help prevent lateral patellar dislocation. Sartorius (6), the longest muscle in the body, passes from the anterior superior iliac spine to the tibia. It flexes and externally rotates the hip, while also flexing the knee to sit cross-legged. The femoral nerve (L2,3,4) supplies all these muscles (knee jerk L3,4). Rectus femoris, crossing two joints, is more susceptible to injury. Quadriceps are essential for knee stability and must not be allowed to waste following joint injury or surgery.

Femoral triangle

The femoral triangle lies between sartorius, the medial border of adductor longus (8) and the inguinal ligament (9). Its floor is formed by the hip flexors iliopsoas (10) and pectineus (11), which is also an adductor, and adductor longus. Its roof is fascia lata. From lateral to medial the triangle contains the femoral nerve (12), artery (13), and vein (14), and the femoral canal. The femoral sheath surrounds only the artery, vein and canal. The latter contains a lymph node and fat. Abdominal contents may pass into the femoral canal as a femoral hernia, visible inferior and lateral to the pubic tubercle.

The femoral artery gives profunda femoris, which sends circumflex femoral arteries and perforating branches to supply the thigh muscles. There are important anastomotic vessels between branches of the femoral arteries and the gluteal arteries. These may provide collateral circulation following occlusion of the femoral artery. The femoral artery and vein pass into the subsartorial canal and through the hiatus in adductor magnus. The femoral pulse is palpable at the mid-inguinal point (this is not the mid-point of the inguinal ligament), midway between the anterior superior iliac spine and the pubic symphysis, and the vein may be accessed just medially.

The femoral nerve (L2,3,4 posterior divisions) passes posterior to the inguinal ligament, and immediately divides into muscular and cutaneous branches. It supplies the skin of the anterior and medial thigh before continuing as the saphenous nerve that passes with the great saphenous vein (15) to supply the skin of the medial leg and medial border of the foot (L4). Both the saphenous nerve and the nerve to vastus medialis pass under sartorius, but neither go through the adductor hiatus.

Lower limb anterior and lateral compartments

In the leg the anterior and lateral compartments contain muscles that arise from the tibia, fibula, interosseous membrane and surrounding fascia. Muscles that pass anterior to the ankle dorsiflex the foot (and toes), whereas those passing behind plantarflex. Muscles that pass medially to attach to the tarsal and metatarsals invert at the subtalar joint and those passing laterally evert. The functional importance is lifting the foot and toes in walking and in keeping the body upright over the foot.

Inversion – Tibialis anterior (22), deep fibular (peroneal) nerve, L4,5.
Dorsiflexion – Tibialis anterior, extensor hallucis longus (23) for the big toe and extensor digitorum longus (24) for the remaining toes. The extensor tendons in the toes form an expansion similar to the fingers. The expansion receives lumbricals, interossei and extensor digitorum brevis (25). The dorsiflexors are supplied by the deep fibular nerve (L4,5).
Eversion (and plantarflexion) – Fibularis longus (26) and brevis (27), superficial fibular nerve (28) (L5,S1).

Damage to the common fibular (peroneal) nerve (L4,5,S1,2), at the fibular neck (car bumper, tight plaster cast) results in foot drop (the foot falls into plantarflexion and inversion). The toes scuff the ground during walking or the leg is lifted high by hip and knee flexion resulting in the foot hitting the ground with a slap. There is sensory loss over the anterolateral leg and dorsum of the foot as the deep fibular supplies the first cleft and the superficial fibular the remainder.

The anterior tibial artery, passing on the interosseous membrane with the deep fibular nerve, comes superficial at the ankle and on the dorsum of the foot it is palpable as the dorsalis pedis pulse (29) between extensors digitorum and hallucis longus.

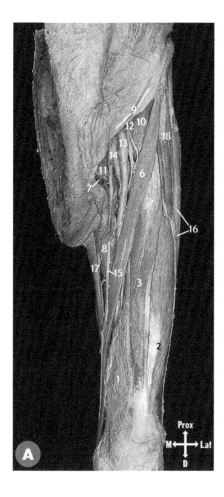

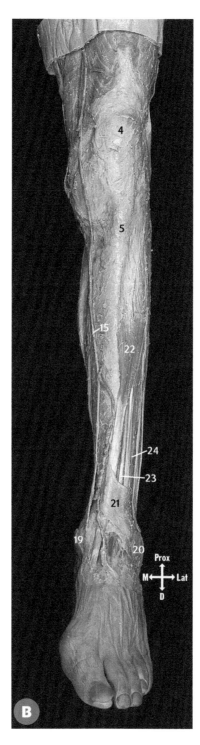

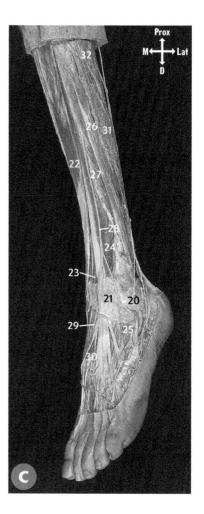

A Left thigh (from the front)
B Left lower limb structures
   (from the front)
C Left lower limb structures
   (from the left)

1	Vastus medialis	9	External oblique aponeurosis
2	Vastus lateralis		becoming inguinal ligament
3	Rectus femoris	10	Iliacus
4	Patella	11	Pectineus
5	Tuberosity of tibia	12	Femoral nerve
6	Sartorius	13	Femoral artery
7	Adductor brevis	14	Femoral vein
8	Adductor longus	15	Great saphenous vein
		16	Iliotibial tract

17	Gracilis
18	Tensor fasciae latae
19	Medial malleolus
20	Lateral malleolus
21	Extensor retinaculum
22	Tibialis anterior
23	Extensor hallucis longus
24	Extensor digitorum longus
25	Extensor digitorum brevis

26	Fibularis (peroneus) longus
27	Fibularis (peroneus) brevis
28	Superficial fibular (peroneal)
	nerve
29	Dorsalis pedis artery
30	Extensor hallucis brevis
31	Soleus
32	Gastrocnemius

Location of numbers: 1A; 2A; 3A 4B; 5B; 6A; 7A; 8A; 9A; 10A; 11A; 12A; 13A; 14A; 15AB; 16A; 17A; 18A; 19B; 20BC; 21BC; 22BC; 23BC; 24BC; 25C;
26C; 27C; 28C; 29C; 30C; 31C; 32C.

Lower limb: posterior muscle groups

The sciatic nerve and its tibial branch supply all the following muscles, which fall into groups for hip extension, knee flexion, ankle and toe plantarflexion, and foot inversion.

Hip extension and knee flexion

The three hamstring muscles lie in the posterior aspect of the thigh, and arise from the ischial tuberosity. Biceps femoris (1) arises from the same tendon as semitendinosus (2), but has a second head from the linea aspera of the femur. It passes to the head of the fibula, its attachment split by the lateral collateral ligament of the knee. Semitendinosus, the lower part of its length being tendon, and semimembranosus (3), the upper part of its length being flat, membranous tendon, pass from the ischial tuberosity to the medial condyle of the tibia.

The hamstrings extend the hip in walking and flex the knee. They pass to either side of the knee joint, therefore, may rotate the flexed knee. As hamstrings cross two joints, they are prone to injury. They are supplied by L5,S1,2 via the sciatic nerve. Therefore, L5,S1,2 are the root values for hip extension and knee flexion.

Knee flexion and ankle plantarflexion

Gastrocnemius (8) is the most superficial, arising by two heads from the femoral condyles, passing into the calf and converging into the calcaneal tendon (9), which inserts into the posterior aspect of the calcaneus. Soleus (10) lies deep to gastrocnemius. It arises from the tibia and fibula and also converges into the calcaneal tendon. The posterior tibial neurovascular bundle lies deep to soleus, which is visible as a linear bulge on the lateral calf in athletes. Gastrocnemius and soleus plantarflex the ankle. Gastrocnemius, because it arises from the femur, also flexes the knee. The tibial nerve (12) (S1,2) supplies both muscles.

Plantaris is a variable muscle arising by a small belly from the lateral femoral condyle and becoming a long, thin tendon lying medial to the calcaneal tendon and inserting into it, or into the calcaneus. It very weakly assists gastrocnemius and has the same nerve supply.

Ankle, toe plantarflexion and inversion

Three muscles lie in the deep compartment and arise from the tibia, fibula and interosseous membrane. They form tendons, which pass in synovial sheaths, deep to a retinaculum behind the medial malleolus (13) where they are accompanied by the posterior tibial neurovascular bundle (14). The posterior tibial pulse is palpable midway between the heel and the medial malleolus.

Tibialis posterior (15) lies immediately next to the tibia and medial malleolus. It inserts into many of the tarsal and metatarsal bones, but mainly the navicular and medial cuneiform. (Tibialis anterior inserts into medial cuneiform and adjacent first metatarsal.) Tibialis posterior is a plantar flexor of the ankle and an invertor of the subtalar joint. Its nerve supply is tibial (L4,5). (Tibialis anterior also not only inverts, but dorsiflexes.) Flexor digitorum longus (16) arises from tibia only and has a tendon lying lateral to that of tibialis posterior as it passes around the ankle to enter the sole and run forward to the distal phalanges. Flexor hallucis longus (17) (mainly from fibula) lies deeply at the ankle, with muscle fibres entering the tendon distally. It passes into the sole and to the distal phalanx of the hallux.

The tibial nerve (S1,2) supplies flexors hallucis and digitorum longus. The actions of all the posterior muscles are important in concert with the anterior and lateral groups, in walking, standing upright and balancing the body over the ankle or angling the foot when walking on uneven ground. Flexor hallucis longus is particularly necessary for the final 'push off' in walking. Ankle and toe plantar flexion are essentially S1,2. The ankle jerk tests S1,2. Inversion is L4,5, whereas eversion is L5,S1.

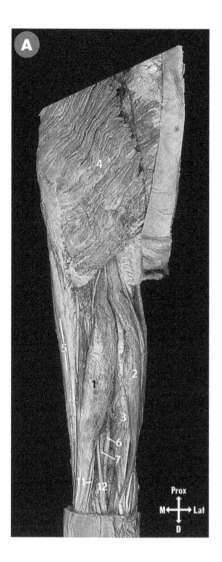

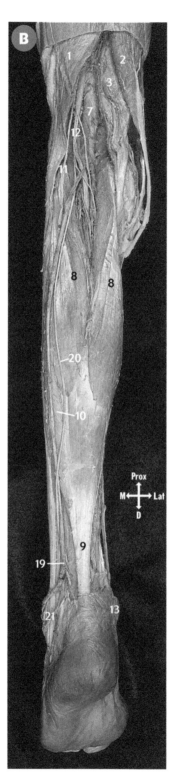

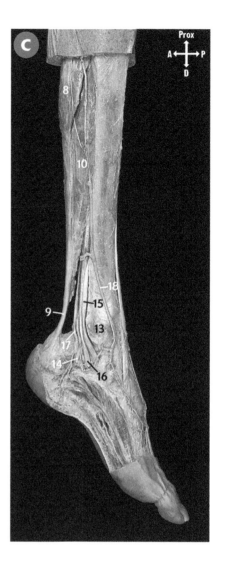

A Left gluteal region (from behind)
B Left lower limb structures (from behind)
C Left leg structures (from the right)

1	Biceps femoris	7	Popliteal vein
2	Semitendinosus	8	Gastrocnemius
3	Semimembranosus	9	Calcaneal (Achilles) tendon
4	Gluteus maximus	10	Soleus
5	Iliotibial tract	11	Common fibular (peroneal) nerve
6	Popliteal artery	12	Tibial nerve

13	Medial malleolus	17	Tendon of flexor hallucis longus
14	Posterior tibial artery and veins, and tibial nerve	18	Great saphenous vein
15	Tendon of tibialis posterior	19	Small saphenous vein
16	Tendon of flexor digitorum longus	20	Sural nerve
		21	Lateral malleolus

Location of numbers: 1AB; 2AB; 3AB; 4A; 5A; 6A; 7AB; 8BC; 9BC; 10BC; 11AB; 12AB; 13BC; 14C; 15C; 16C; 17C; 18C; 19B; 20B; 21B.

Buttock musculature, sciatic nerve

In the buttock, the sacrum (1) is medial, the greater trochanter (2) lateral, and midway between the two is the prominent ischial tuberosity (3). Structures passing medial to the tuberosity, between it and the sacrum, are passing to the perineum. Structures passing lateral to the tuberosity, between it and the greater trochanter are passing to the posterior thigh.

Hip extension

The rounded shape of the buttock is created by subcutaneous fat overlying the musculature. The region is divided (left, right) by the natal cleft. Gluteus maximus (4) arises from the posterior part of the ilium, the sacrum and sacrotuberous ligament (5). It inserts into the gluteal tuberosity to provide powerful hip extension when running, climbing stairs and standing from sitting. Maximus also inserts into the iliotibial tract (6) with tensor fasciae latae. Consequently it supports the knee close-packed in extension and helps gluteus medius and minimus hold the pelvis level during walking. The iliotibial tract turns the lower limb into a strong, supportive strut for the body. Maximus is supplied by the inferior gluteal vessels and nerve (7) (L5,S1,2). There is a bursa allowing movement between it and the ischial tuberosity.

Hip abduction

Gluteus medius (8) and minimus (9) arise deep to maximus, from the lateral aspect of the ilium. Minimus is covered by medius. Both insert onto the lateral aspect of the greater trochanter, medius posteriorly and minimus anteriorly. Both muscles are powerful abductors of the hip but their important function is to work in concert with the adductors and the iliotibial tract to prevent pelvic tilt during walking. Medius and minimus, along with tensor fasciae latae are supplied by the superior gluteal vessels and nerve (10) (L4,5,S1).

Hip lateral rotation

Inferomedial to gluteus medius, piriformis (11) passes from the inner aspect of the sacrum, to the tip of the greater trochanter. Obturator internus (12), from the internal aspect of the obturator membrane, and obturator externus, from the external aspect of the membrane, pass to the medial aspect of the greater trochanter. Internus has the superior (13) and inferior (14) gemelli lying parallel to its tendon. Quadratus femoris (15) passes from the ischial tuberosity to the quadrate tubercle on the intertrochanteric crest of the femur.

All these muscles pass behind the hip joint therefore laterally rotate it. When the lower limb swings forward during walking, so does the pelvis on the same side. Lateral rotation of the femur ensures that the lower limb and foot are pointing forward. Branches of the lumbosacral plexus, ranging from L4 to S2 supply the muscles.

Nerves in the buttock

There are a number of small, named nerves within the buttock, passing to the overlying skin of the buttock and the perineum. They are branches of the gluteal nerves and lumbosacral plexus and their root values range from L4 to S4. The posterior femoral cutaneous (16), (S1,2,3) supplies branches to the perineum, and skin of the posterior thigh to just below the knee.

The sciatic nerve (17) (L4,5,S1,2,3) is formed within the pelvis from L4,5 (the lumbosacral trunk), and the ventral rami of S1,2,3. It emerges into the buttock via the greater sciatic foramen, usually inferior to piriformis and passes into the thigh. As it does so, the sciatic lies posterior to the hip joint, then midway between the ischial tuberosity and the greater trochanter. Intramuscular injections must be given in the superolateral quadrant of the buttock, well away from the sciatic nerve.

The nerve passes deep to biceps femoris (18), to lie buried between it and semitendinosus (19). It supplies the hamstrings and also sends a branch to adductor magnus (20), augmenting the latter's supply from the obturator nerve. In the popliteal fossa the sciatic divides into tibial (21) and common fibular (22) branches. The site of the division is very variable, occurring anywhere between the buttock and the popliteal fossa.

The tibial nerve (L4,5,S1,2,3 anterior divisions) passes inferiorly more or less in the middle of the popliteal fossa, superficial to the artery and vein. It passes deep to gastrocnemius and soleus, which it supplies and runs with the posterior tibial artery in the fascial septum that separates the superficial from the deep muscular compartment.

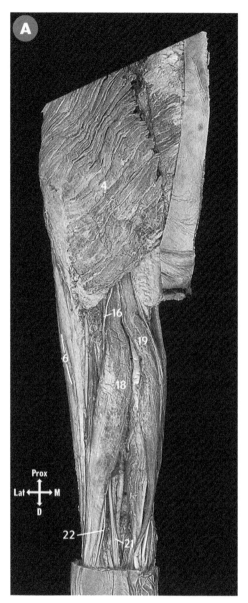

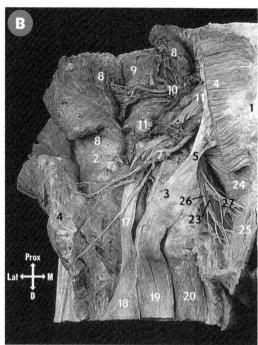

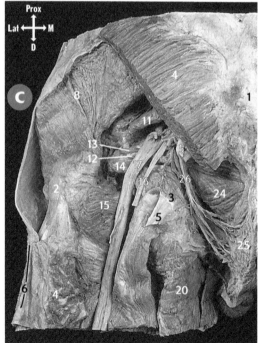

A Left gluteal region (from behind)
B Left gluteal region (from behind)
C Left gluteal region (from behind)

1	Sacrum	8	Gluteus medius	15	Quadratus femoris	22	Common fibular (peroneal)
2	Greater trochanter of femur	9	Gluteus minimus	16	Posterior femoral cutaneous		nerve
3	Ischial tuberosity	10	Superior gluteal artery, vein and		nerve	23	Internal pudendal artery
4	Gluteus maximus		nerve	17	Sciatic nerve	24	Levator ani
5	Sacrotuberous ligament	11	Piriformis	18	Biceps femoris	25	External anal sphincter
6	Iliotibial tract	12	Obturator internus	19	Semitendinosus	26	Pudendal nerve
7	Inferior gluteal artery, vein and	13	Superior gemellus	20	Adductor magnus	27	Inferior rectal artery, vein and
	nerve	14	Inferior gemellus	21	Tibial nerve		nerve

Location of numbers: 1BC; 2BC; 3BC; 4ABC; 5BC; 6ABC; 7B; 8BC; 9B; 10B; 11BC; 12C; 13C; 14C; 15C; 16AC; 17BC; 18AB; 19AB; 20BC; 21A; 22A; 23B; 24BC; 25BC; 26BC; 27B.

Appendix to abdomen and pelvis: structures and concepts not visible on illustrations

Blood vessels

The abdominal aorta passes behind the median arcuate ligament of the diaphragm at the level of T12. It supplies the undersurface of the diaphragm via the inferior phrenic arteries that also send superior suprarenal arteries to the suprarenal gland. The aorta gives the middle suprarenal arteries, whereas the inferior suprarenals arise from the renal arteries. Lumbar arteries arise from the aorta to supply the abdominal wall, and they also send spinal arteries through the intervertebral foramina to augment the blood supply to the spinal cord. **Occlusion of these may cause cord ischaemia.**

The coeliac trunk (axis) arises at the level of T12 and supplies the structures derived from the embryological foregut. The superior mesenteric artery (SMA) arises at L1 to supply structures derived from the midgut. The left and right renal arteries to the kidneys and adrenals arise at L2, with the gonadal arteries arising just below. The inferior mesenteric artery (IMA), to hindgut derived structures, arises at L3. The aorta divides at L4 into the common iliac arteries.

The coeliac trunk arises from the front of the aorta, between the diaphragmatic crura, above the pancreas and behind the lesser sac. It divides into the left gastric, splenic and (common) hepatic arteries. The left gastric artery passes on the diaphragm to where the oesophagus pierces it. The artery divides and sends a branch up through the diaphragm to anastomose with the oesophageal branches from the thoracic aorta to supply the lower third of the oesophagus. The left gastric continues into the lesser omentum to run along the lesser curvature of the stomach. The splenic artery takes a tortuous course behind the pancreas, and passes with it, in the lienorenal ligament, to supply the spleen. It sends short gastrics in the gastrosplenic ligament to supply the fundus of the stomach, the left gastro-epiploic to supply the greater curvature of the stomach and greater omentum, and the greater pancreatic artery to the pancreas. The (common) hepatic artery passes to the right, lifts off the posterior abdominal wall to enter the free edge of the lesser omentum and passes to the liver as the hepatic artery. The (common) hepatic gives the right gastric and the gastroduodenal. The latter divides into the right gastro-epiploic and the superior pancreaticoduodenal.

There is an anastomotic ring of vessels around the stomach, and free anastomosis in the duodenum between branches of the coeliac trunk and SMA. The SMA arises behind the pancreas and (with its vein) passes between the neck and uncinate process of the pancreas, anterior to the duodenum (third part), behind the transverse mesocolon and into the mesentery to supply the midgut. It supplies the pancreas and duodenum via the inferior pancreaticoduodenal artery and the transverse colon via the middle colic. In the mesentery the SMA gives jejunal and ileal branches to form arcades within the mesentery. Near its termination it sends right colic arteries to the ascending colon, and the ileocolic to the ileum, caecum and appendix. The appendicular artery arises from the posterior caecal branch of the ileocolic.

The IMA passes to the left, behind the peritoneum to supply the hindgut. It sends left colic and sigmoid branches to the descending and sigmoid colon. It ends as the superior rectal that passes into the pelvis to anastomose with the middle and inferior rectal arteries and supply the rectum and anal canal. Within the curve of the large bowel, the right colic, middle colic and left colic arteries anastomose with each other to form the marginal artery. **Slow occlusion of the IMA by an aortic aneurysm allows a collateral circulation to open via the marginal artery.**

The inferior mesenteric vein is the continuation of the superior rectal vein from the rectum and anal canal. They are also drained by middle and inferior rectal veins to the internal iliac, therefore the lower rectum and anal canal are sites of portosystemic anastomosis. The inferior mesenteric vein passes up the posterior abdominal wall, medial to the left gonadal vein and ureter. It usually enters the splenic vein, behind the pancreas, but may enter the superior mesenteric vein or the portal vein directly.

Lymph nodes and vessels lie on the anterior and lateral surfaces of the aorta. These converge to form the cisterna chyli that passes behind the median arcuate ligament (to the right of the aorta), to continue as the thoracic duct. The part of the gastrointestinal tract supplied by a particular artery sends lymph back to the nodes on the aorta around that artery.

Autonomic innervation

The splanchnic nerves arise from the sympathetic trunk in the thorax and pass through the crura of the diaphragm to converge on a plexus of nerves and ganglia around the coeliac trunk, SMA and IMA. The greater splanchnic (T5–9) synapses in the coeliac ganglia, to be distributed with branches of the coeliac trunk to all foregut structures. The lesser splanchnic (T10,11) synapses in the superior mesenteric ganglia, to be distributed with the SMA to all the midgut, as well as to the gonads via the gonadal arteries. The least splanchnic (T12) synapses in the inferior mesenteric ganglia to be distributed to the hindgut with branches of the IMA.

Below the IMA the plexus continues downward on the front of the aorta as the pre-aortic plexus. The plexus is augmented by lumbar splanchnics, which arise in the L1,2 segments of the cord, and which emerge from the lumbar part of the sympathetic trunk. The pre-aortic plexus passes over the pelvic brim as the superior hypogastric nerve and divides into the left and right pelvic plexuses or inferior hypogastric nerves. Sympathetic (thoracolumbar) innervation is generally to slow down intestinal function by shutting sphincters and decreasing peristalsis, to divert energy for 'fight or flight'.

Parasympathetic (craniosacral) efferents are to promote digestive function by opening sphincters and increasing peristalsis. These are from the vagus nerves, which enter the abdomen with the oesophagus and are distributed as far as two-thirds along the transverse colon via the coeliac and superior mesenteric plexuses. The hindgut receives parasympathetic innervation

arising from S2–4 and passing via the pelvic plexuses, up the superior hypogastric nerve to reach the inferior mesenteric plexus, for distribution with the IMA.

Referred pain

The sympathetic nerves all have afferent fibres running with them. These transmit the signals of visceral pain and distension back to the cord segments from which they arise. The brain cannot localize visceral pain and perceives it as arising from the skin of the equivalent dermatome in the midline i.e. visceral, referred pain.

All foregut pain refers to the epigastrium, i.e. the T5–9 dermatomes. Midgut (including appendix) and gonadal pain refers to the T10,11 dermatomes around the umbilicus. An embryological remnant, Meckel's diverticulum, is said to be 5 cm (two inches) long and occurs in two-thirds of people and originates 0.6 m (two feet) from the end of the ileum. It may become inflamed and the pain mimics that of appendicitis. Hindgut pain refers to the T12 dermatome that is suprapubic. Once an inflamed or distended viscus affects the overlying parietal peritoneum, the pain is localized, as the parietal peritoneum is sensitive and supplied by the same nerves that supply the overlying skin.

Inguinal canal

During embryonic development the testis migrates down the posterior abdominal wall, through the anterior wall and into the scrotum. It carries the vas, the testicular neurovascular supply and the processus vaginalis (an extension of the peritoneal cavity) with it. The tunnel through the anterior abdominal wall remains as the inguinal canal. In the female it transmits the round ligament of the uterus.

In the male the testis, vas and testicular vessels 'pick up' the layers of spermatic fascia that form the spermatic cord as they pass the abdominal fascia and muscles. Transversalis fascia provides the internal spermatic fascia. The conjoint tendon provides the cremaster muscle and cremasteric fascia. The external oblique muscle provides the external spermatic fascia to complete the spermatic cord as it leaves the abdomen. The terminal branches of the ilio-inguinal nerve commence deep to the external spermatic fascia.

The cremaster muscle receives the artery to cremaster (from the inferior epigastric) and its sympathetic nerve supply is with the genital branch of the genitofemoral nerve (L1,2) that reaches it via the deep inguinal ring. Cremaster helps dartos retract the testis. The cremaster reflex is mediated by L1 and is testicular retraction following stroking of the skin on the upper medial thigh.

The spermatic cord, comprising the three layers of spermatic fascia, contains:

- vas deferens with its artery to the vas, derived from the inferior vesical.
- testicular artery, from the aorta at L2, and carrying sympathetic efferents, and afferents derived from the lesser splanchnic nerve (T10,11) to the testis.
- pampiniform plexus of veins that coalesces to form the testicular vein. The left testicular vein drains, at right angles, into the left renal vein and this may cause a varicocele, a tortuous dilatation of the pampiniform plexus, visible and palpable through the scrotal skin. Left-sided varicoceles also raise the suspicion of left-sided renal tumours that have invaded the renal vein.

Testicular lymph drainage is to the para-aortic nodes. Therefore testicular tumours will spread to these para-aortic nodes. The inguinal nodes are only involved if the testicular tumour spreads to the scrotum.

The inguinal canal tunnels through, or under the abdominal-wall muscles ensuring that the two openings of the tunnel, the deep and superficial rings, are supported and protected by two of the muscles. The deep inguinal ring is just above the mid-point of the inguinal ligament, midway between the pubic tubercle and anterior superior iliac spine. The femoral artery passes below the inguinal ligament a little medially at the mid-inguinal point, midway between the pubic symphysis and the anterior superior iliac spine. The deep ring is an opening in the transversalis fascia. It lies just lateral to the inferior epigastric artery and just medial to the lowest fibres of transversus abdominis as they arise from the inguinal ligament and curve over the canal, to form its roof, then its posterior wall, as the conjoint tendon. (Opinions differ on the position of the deep ring and some authors place it at the mid-inguinal point.)

The aponeurosis of external oblique and the muscle fibres of internal oblique are anterior to the deep ring. Half to two-thirds of the way along the inguinal liga-

ment the internal oblique fibres then curve over the canal, to contribute to its roof and then to its posterior wall as the conjoint tendon. The superficial (external) ring is a triangular opening in the external oblique aponeurosis. The base is on the pubic crest. The apex is above and lateral to the pubic tubercle. The edges of the 'ring' are the medial and lateral crura, supported where they meet at the apex of the triangle by intercrural fibres of external oblique aponeurosis. The conjoint tendon, as it attaches to the pubic crest and pecten lies behind the superficial ring, to protect and support it.

The inguinal canal has:

- A floor – inguinal ligament
- A roof – transversus abdominis and internal oblique
- An anterior wall – external and internal oblique laterally, only external oblique medially
- A posterior wall – transversalis fascia laterally, both internal oblique and transversus abdominis, fused as the conjoint tendon, medially.

Scrotum

In the scrotum, the testis, epididymis and vas appear to invaginate into an extension of the peritoneal cavity, the tunica vaginalis from behind so that a visceral layer of mesothelium covers them. Posteriorly, in the spermatic cord, this visceral layer reflects to become the parietal layer, leaving an intervening potential space with a little serous fluid. Initially, in the infant, this potential space communicates with the peritoneal cavity, but that connection should obliterate completely to leave the processus vaginalis in the spermatic cord. If it does not obliterate, abdominal contents may herniate into the processus and consequently into the scrotum. Partial obliteration may leave cysts.

The parietal layer is itself surrounded by the three layers of spermatic fascia. The parietal layer of tunica vaginalis and the three spermatic fascias of each testis fuse in the middle of the scrotum to form a septum. Consequently, the testis is effectively suspended in the scrotum, within a potential space between the parietal and visceral layers of the tunica vaginalis. Occasionally the testis may rotate within this space, twisting and therefore compromising the blood supply. This condition, torsion of the testis, must be recognized and surgically treated within about five hours, before the testis becomes necrotic. The potential space within the tunica vaginalis may fill with fluid, a hydrocele. Embryological remnants leave little appendices on the epididymis and upper pole of the testis. These may become painfully inflamed.

Superficial fascia of the penis and scrotum

Penile superficial fascia has a membranous inner layer (Buck's fascia) that is continuous with Scarpa's fascia in the lower anterior abdominal wall and upper thigh. Posteriorly, this fascia is continuous with the superficial fascia of the scrotum (Colles') that attaches to the pubic bones, ischiopubic rami, and perineal body in the midline, just anterior to the anal opening. This superficial fascia forms the superficial boundary of the superficial perineal pouch.

Pelvic fractures and/or urethral rupture may cause bleeding and extravasation of urine that is held within the fascial space deep to this membranous layer of fascia. The consequent bruising is visible on the lower abdomen, upper thighs, penis and scrotum, but stopping just anterior to the anus.

Hernias

Weaknesses in the anterior abdominal wall may allow the development of a hernia, which is prolapse or extrusion of abdominal contents, from small tags of fat, to loops of bowel.

Inguinal hernias appear at the superficial ring above the pubic tubercle. They may enter the scrotum.
- Indirect inguinal – usually in young males, sometimes with a patent processus vaginalis. The hernia passes into the deep ring, lateral to the inferior epigastric artery, and down the inguinal canal. Once reduced, such hernias maybe controlled by the examining surgeon applying pressure on the skin over the site of the deep ring.
- Direct inguinal – occurring as a result of general weakness in the abdominal muscles or conjoint tendon. The hernia pushes into the inguinal canal, straight through the posterior wall, or pushing the posterior wall in advance of it. It occurs in the inguinal triangle, bounded inferiorly by the inguinal ligament, laterally by the inferior epigastric artery and medially by the lateral edge of rectus abdominis. Consequently a direct hernia is medial to the inferior epigastric artery, whereas an indirect hernia is lateral. The fibres of internal oblique and transversus abdominis that form the conjoint tendon are supplied by the iliohypogastric nerve (L1). This nerve may be injured during appendicectomy, possibly leading to a weakness of the conjoint tendon and consequent inguinal herniation.

Umbilical hernias. The umbilicus is the puckered scar left on the abdominal wall by the embryonic umbilical cord that contained the umbilical vein and arteries, the urachus and the vitello-intestinal duct. Hernias may extrude through the umbilicus or just to one side of it (para-umbilical).

Incisional hernias follow failure of muscle closure post operatively. Every attempt is made when incising the abdomen to prevent damage to the neurovascular supply and to avoid cutting muscle fibres. The preferred route is to separate the muscle fibres in their direction. Incisions through the avascular linea alba may facilitate rapid access, but healing may be difficult due to that avascularity. Paramedian incisions are through the rectus sheath, and then reflecting rectus abdominis.

Femoral hernias are more common in the female, with the wider pelvis, and are through the femoral canal, between the lacunar ligament and femoral vein, posterior to the inguinal ligament. They appear below and lateral to the pubic tubercle and are more likely to incarcerate.

Lumbar hernias occur posteriorly (and very rarely) in the triangle between the free posterior edge of external oblique, latissimus dorsi and the iliac crest.

Pelvic peritoneum

The peritoneum dips inferiorly from the abdomen to cover the organs in the pelvis, creating a continuous abdominopelvic, peritoneal cavity. From anterior to posterior the peritoneum covers the bladder, then the uterus and uterine (Fallopian) tubes with the vesico-uterine pouch between, and then the rectum, with the recto-uterine pouch between. The peritoneum passes down the anterior abdominal wall, onto the superior and posterior surfaces of the bladder. As a result the bladder is inferior to the peritoneal cavity and as it fills it extends upward, pushing the peritoneum upward with it.

Urinary obstruction (usually caused by prostatic hypertrophy in the male) causes the bladder to extend up into the abdomen. It always pushes the peritoneum and the organs within the peritoneal cavity upward and behind it, so that the bladder lies immediately posterior to the anterior abdominal wall. If necessary, a suprapubic catheter may be safely passed through the abdominal wall, just above the pubic symphysis, and into the bladder to drain it.

The recto-uterine pouch (of Douglas) is the lowest point in the abdominopelvic cavity. Blood, fluid or pus may descend into it. At this point the peritoneum lies on the upper, posterior aspect of the vagina, its posterior fornix. The recto-uterine pouch may be surgically drained via the vagina. But instruments used ineptly in abortions may pierce the posterior fornix and enter the peritoneal cavity, possibly introducing severe infection.

In either sex, the lower third of the rectum lies completely outside the peritoneal cavity and does not have peritoneum on it at all. But peritoneum clothes the anterior surface of its middle third, and the anterior surface and sides of its upper third.

Pelvic ligaments (female)

The uterine tubes have the appearance of having pushed upward into the peritoneal cavity to create a fold of peritoneum with anterior and posterior layers that pass laterally to reach the pelvic wall. The two layers form the broad ligament. The anterior layer continues as the peritoneum on the anterior abdominal wall. The posterior layer continues as the peritoneum on the posterior abdominal wall. As a result, the ovarian neurovascular bundle passes down the posterior abdominal wall and enters the lateral aspect of the broad ligament to create the suspensory ligament of the ovary.

In the embryo, the ovary forms on the posterior abdominal wall, and migrates into the pelvis, guided by the gubernaculum, which remains as the ligament of the ovary and the round ligament of the uterus. The round ligament of the uterus passes laterally from the uterus, in the broad ligament, to reach the anterior

abdominal wall and enter the deep inguinal ring. It is thought to hold the uterus in its normal anteverted and anteflexed position. The ligament of the ovary attaches the ovary to the side wall of uterus.

In the female, as the ovary is truly intraperitoneal and the ovum is secreted into the peritoneal cavity, the infundibulum pierces the posterior leaf of the broad ligament so that the fimbriae overhang the ovary in the peritoneal cavity. This anatomical arrangement means that in the female, the peritoneal cavity is effectively open to the exterior via the vagina, uterus and uterine tubes. Foreign matter may enter the peritoneal cavity by this route. To prevent this, the epithelium and mucous membrane of the tube are highly folded and the folds interdigitate with each other. The uterine cavity is very narrow and mucous membrane folds in the cervix also interdigitate with each other. The anterior and posterior walls of the vagina are normally opposed to each other. Rarely, it is possible to override this protective, safety mechanism.

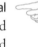

Anal continence and defecation

Faeces remains in the sigmoid colon before descending into the rectum where its distending presence is detected by afferents in the parasympathetic system and the desire to defecate is initiated.

The circular layer of smooth muscle in the wall of the intestinal tract thickens as the internal anal sphincter that is under autonomic control and ends at the white line (intersphincteric groove). The puborectalis portion of levator ani sweeps around the recto-anal junction. Its contraction pulls the junction forward, making the angle between the rectum and anal canal more acute, helping to hold faeces in the rectum. The external anal sphincter, of striated muscle, encircles the anal canal, in three parts, the deep, superficial and subcutaneous. The superficial part not only encircles the anal canal like the others, but also attaches to the anococcygeal ligament and the perineal body.

Fibres of puborectalis fuse with fibres of the deep part of the external sphincter and with fibres of the internal sphincter to form the anorectal ring, which is necessary for continence and is palpable on rectal examination. During defecation puborectalis and the external sphincter relax under the influence of the perineal branches of S3,4 and the inferior rectal branches of the pudendal nerve (S2,3,4). The colon contracts and the internal sphincter relaxes, under parasympathetic control that also arises from S2,3,4. The abdominal wall is voluntarily contracted to raise the intra-abdominal pressure.

Micturition, erection and ejaculation

The bladder fills by paying-out under the parasympathetic control of detrusor. Usually at about 310 mL there is a desire to micturate. The sensation is carried mainly by parasympathetic afferents, but painful stimuli are via sympathetics.

With simultaneous contraction of the abdominal wall, the parasympathetic supply via the pelvic splanchnics (S2,3,4) causes detrusor contraction and urine enters the urethra. In the male, the sympathetic supply to the internal urethral sphincter is over-ridden, so it relaxes. The sensation of urine in the urethra is via the pudendal nerve (S2,3,4) and this sensation maintains the micturition reflex. This is an example of involuntary and voluntary reflexes working together at S2,3,4.

During erection, the parasympathetic system is also said to over-ride the sympathetic supply to the penile arteries, causing them to dilate and the penis to become erect. But at ejaculation the sympathetic takes over causing some contraction of the muscular components of the reproductive ducts and closure of the internal urethral sphincter to prevent backflow of semen to the bladder. The pudendal nerve and its branches contain sympathetic fibres from the pelvic plexus, and parasympathetic fibres from the sacral splanchnics (S2,3,4). Erection is under parasympathetic control, but ejaculation is sympathetic.

Bibliography

Books

Ellis H, Logan BM, Dixon AK (1999) *Human Sectional Anatomy: Atlas Of Body Sections, CT and MRI Images*. 2nd edn. Oxford: Butterworth-Heinemann.

Federative Committee on Anatomical Terminology (1998) *Terminologia Anatomica – International Anatomical Terminology*. Stuttgart: Thieme.

Logan BM, Reynolds P, Hutchings RT (2004) *McMinn's Colour Atlas of Head and Neck Anatomy*, 3rd edn. London: Mosby.

Logan BM, Singh D, Hutchings RT (2004) *McMinn's Colour Atlas of Foot and Ankle Anatomy*, 3rd edn. London: Mosby.

McMinn RMH, Gaddum-Rosse P, Hutchings RT, Logan BM (1995) *McMinn's Functional and Clinical Anatomy*. London: Mosby-Wolfe.

Moore K, Dalley AF (1999) *Clinically Orientated Anatomy*, 4th edn. Baltimore, MD: Lippincott, Williams & Wilkins.

Romanes GJ (ed) (1981) *Cunningham's Textbook of Anatomy*, 12th edn. Oxford: Oxford University Press.

Sinnatamby CS (ed) (1999) *Last's Anatomy Regional and Applied*, 10th edn. Edinburgh: Churchill Livingstone.

Standring S (ed) (2005) *Gray's Anatomy*, 39th edn. London: Elsevier Churchill Livingstone.

Other resources

Dyball R (Cambridge), Davies CD (St George's), McHanwell S (Newcastle), Morris JF (Oxford), Parkin IG (Cambridge), Whiten S (St Andrew's), Wilton J (Birmingham). Setting a benchmark for anatomical knowledge and its assessment (A core curriculum for the teaching of anatomy to medical students, available at: www.anatsoc.org.uk).

Bridger John (2006) Revision anatomy for clinical students. Cambridge: Department of Anatomy, University of Cambridge.

Index

The majority of references are to core structures. Page numbers are almost all for left hand (text) pages of each double page spread. Readers can assume that they will find the structure on the facing right hand (illustrated) page. Non-core anatomical structures have generally not been indexed. The exception is to the appendix section (on abdominal and pelvic structures and concepts not visible in illustrations) and these page numbers are in italics.

Printed and bound by CPI Group (UK) Ltd, Croydon, CR0 4YY

23/10/2024

01778251-0018